Wall Pilates Workouts for Women

Emily Lemberg

Disclaimer:

The information and exercises this book outlines are intended for educational purposes, not as a substitute for professional medical guidance or treatment. The author is not a healthcare practitioner, and the contents of this book should not be perceived as professional medical advice, diagnosis, or treatment. Always consult your doctor or a qualified healthcare provider before embarking on any new fitness program or modifying an existing one.

The author and publisher shall not be held accountable for any injuries, health conditions, or adverse effects that may occur as a result of applying the methods described in this book. The responsibility for health and safety remains entirely with the reader.

DEDICATION

To every woman who faces challenges head-on, finds strength in adversity, and carves out moments for self-care in the hustle of life. This one's for you.

Table of Contents

Introduction

Are you frustrated with fitness routines that seem out of sync with your body's needs and abilities? Are traditional workouts leaving you exhausted, bored, or even hurt? Do you find yourself constantly searching for an exercise regimen that resonates with your unique physical needs as a woman and fosters mental well-being? If you're nodding in agreement, you've turned the page to the right book.

Welcome to Wall Pilates, your gateway to an empowering and transformative fitness journey. A unique fusion of traditional Pilates principles with the stability of a wall, Wall Pilates is designed to resonate with women's specific needs. Imagine exercises that strengthen your core, enhance your posture, increase your flexibility, and build your mind-body connection. Now envision these benefits translating into your daily life, affecting everything from walking, working, sleeping, and interacting with the world around you.

But this book continues beyond just promising these benefits. Instead, it guides you on how to attain them. As an experienced Wall Pilates instructor, I've seen firsthand the transformative power of this fitness approach. In this6 book, I share my professional insights, providing practical and easy-to-follow exercises, strategies, and tips to help you fully embrace Wall Pilates. From setting up your own Wall Pilates space at home to mastering various routines, every chapter is designed to usher you one step closer to your fitness goals.

By turning the last page, you won't just be familiar with Wall Pilates; you'll have incorporated it into your lifestyle. You will stand taller, move with grace, and radiate a new-found inner strength, a testament to your Wall Pilates journey.

So, are you ready to turn the frustrations of past workout disappointments into a rewarding path toward health and well-being? Let's begin this transformative journey together. In Chapter 1, we'll demystify Wall Pilates, illustrating its unique appeal, especially for women. You're just one step away from redefining fitness - let's dive in!

Chapter 1: Why Wall Pilates?

In the complex symphony of modern life, women often play multiple instruments at once. Balancing work, family, and personal time can leave little room for regular exercise. Yet, during these hectic times, self-care becomes even more critical. Enter Wall Pilates, a form of exercise that addresses the body and mind and is adaptable to any lifestyle. As your guide and mentor on this journey, I support you in taking control of your fitness and well-being in a way that fits seamlessly into your life.

Benefits of Wall Pilates for Women

Wall Pilates offers a unique blend of strength, flexibility, and mental clarity. It is a form of exercise that allows you to build a strong core, improve your posture, and enhance your overall physique - all elements that can significantly impact your confidence and self-esteem. More than just a physical workout, Wall Pilates fosters a mindful connection between your body and mind, providing a refreshing mental break amid the chaos of everyday life.

How Wall Pilates Differs from Traditional Pilates

Wall Pilates and traditional Pilates focus on core strength, flexibility, and the mind-body connection. However, Wall Pilates has a unique edge - it uses a wall as a prop, offering a novel way to modify and intensify exercises to cater to all fitness levels. This innovative approach allows beginners to maintain stability and focus on form and alignment while providing a new layer of challenge for advanced practitioners.

Addressing Common Concerns and Misconceptions

When venturing into new fitness territory, it's natural to encounter doubts and apprehensions. Some may wonder if Wall Pilates can provide a comprehensive workout or if it carries a risk of injury. In this guide, I aim to debunk such misconceptions. Wall Pilates is not only a safe but also a highly effective form of exercise. By emphasizing the correct form and technique, we can minimize the risk of injury while maximizing the benefits.

My goal is more than just to provide you with a list of exercises. Instead, I want to empower you with knowledge and skills to adapt Wall Pilates to your unique needs and progress at your own pace. This journey concerns your need to feel stronger, healthier, and more balanced.

As we close this chapter, let me leave you with a piece of motivation from the renowned Pilates instructor, Romana Kryzanowska, who said, "*Pilates is complete coordination of body, mind, and spirit.*" With Wall Pilates, you are on the verge of an empowering journey that will bring harmony to these three aspects of your being.

In the next chapter, "Foundations of Wall Pilates," we will delve deeper into the origins and principles of Pilates and Wall Pilates, further equipping you with the knowledge you need to make the most of this journey. So, let's turn the page and continue on this path to a healthier, stronger you.

Chapter 2: Foundations of Wall Pilates

Welcome to the second chapter of our exploration into Wall Pilates. Before we explore the 'how' behind Wall Pilates, let's explore its history. After all, understanding where something comes from can enhance our appreciation of it. Following this brief historical detour, we'll discuss the foundational principles of Pilates and how they translate into Wall Pilates. As your guide, I promise to help you establish a deep understanding, forming a solid groundwork for your Wall Pilates journey.

Origins of Wall Pilates

Pilates, at its heart, is a form of exercise that focuses on balance, strength, flexibility, and awareness to support physical and mental well-being. Joseph Pilates created it in the early 20th century when the material fitness culture we know today began taking shape.

However, Wall Pilates is a more recent development. It emerged out of a desire to make Pilates more accessible and adaptable. Using a wall as a prop is not unique to Pilates - it's also seen in yoga and other fitness disciplines. But in the context of Pilates, it provides the added stability and orientation that help make the exercises more manageable, especially for beginners.

The introduction of Wall Pilates has opened up new possibilities, especially for those who might find floor or reformer Pilates challenging. It has also added a new dimension to Pilates workouts, providing an opportunity to deepen and expand the practice.

Understanding Pilates Principles

Pilates is founded on six essential principles - Breath, Alignment, Centering, Control, Precision, and Flow. Each one plays a critical role in every movement and transition in Pilates, contributing to the effectiveness of this method in transforming body and mind.

Breath, Alignment, Centering, Control, Precision, Flow.

Breath: Deep and rhythmic breathing oxygenates your muscles, focuses your mind, and energizes your movements.

Alignment: Maintaining proper alignment ensures balanced muscle development, enhances joint health, and mitigates the risk of injury.

Centering: By concentrating on the 'powerhouse' or the core, you cultivate a robust and stable center that supports all other movements.

Control: This principle emphasizes quality over quantity or speed, ensuring that you're using the right muscles, maintaining appropriate form, and protecting yourself from injury.

Precision: Precision goes hand-in-hand with control. It's about performing each movement with care and attention, enhancing body awareness and coordination over time.

Flow: By connecting your movements flowingly, you bring an element of grace and efficiency to your workouts, making the exercise feel more like a dance than a drill.

How the Principles Apply to Wall Pilates

Wall Pilates adheres faithfully to these principles while offering a new dimension of support and challenge. The wall, acting as a tactile reference, assists with alignment, control, and precision and encourages smooth, flowing movements.

Creating a Mind-Body Connection

Wall Pilates is not just about the physical workout - it's about fostering mindfulness and enhancing your connection with your body. This connection allows you to tune into your body, becoming more aware of its signals and modifying your workouts accordingly.

As we wrap up this chapter, let's remember these words from Joseph Pilates, "*Physical fitness is the first requisite of happiness*." Your dedication to understanding these foundational principles is a significant step towards achieving physical fitness and a happier, healthier life.

We'll transition into the next chapter now, where we'll talk about setting up your space and choosing the right equipment for Wall Pilates. We aim to provide you with a practical guide to ensure your safety and maximize the effectiveness of your workouts. So, let's turn the page and continue this empowering journey.

Chapter 3: Essential Equipment and Space Setup for Wall Pilates

Welcome to the next exciting chapter of your Wall Pilates journey. Now that you understand the philosophy and principles of Wall Pilates, you're ready to take your first steps into actual practice. However, preparing the right environment and having the necessary equipment on hand is crucial before you begin. This chapter will guide you through the minimum requirements, ideal space setup, equipment selection, and fundamental safety guidelines for practicing Wall Pilates.

Minimal Requirements for Wall Pilates

One of the critical benefits of Wall Pilates is its simplicity and accessibility. Compared to other forms of exercise, Wall Pilates doesn't demand a significant investment in equipment or expansive space. All you need is a sturdy, flat wall with enough space to extend your arms and legs in all directions freely. Ensure this area is clean, free from any obstacles, and provides a safe space for movement. Prioritize your safety and comfort – the foundation of an enjoyable and practical Wall Pilates experience.

Setting Up a Dedicated Wall Pilates Space

Having a dedicated practice space is advantageous to maximize the benefits of Wall Pilates. Locate a quiet and private area in your home where you won't be disturbed and where you can focus solely on your exercises. A dedicated space will help condition your mind and body, reinforcing your commitment and consistency. To enhance the ambiance, consider adding some personal touches. Plants, calming colors, soft lighting, or a peaceful photograph can transform your exercise corner into a unique sanctuary for physical and mental well-being.

Choosing the Right Equipment and Accessories

While Wall Pilates primarily leverages your body and the wall, incorporating additional accessories can optimize your practice. A top-quality yoga or Pilates mat ensures comfort and prevents potential slips. Grip socks can also be a beneficial addition, offering extra stability and reducing the risk of sliding. While some enthusiasts opt to use resistance bands or Pilates balls to add an element of strength and stabilization, these are not essential for this book's exercises. The beauty of Wall Pilates lies in its simplicity and accessibility, with your body playing the starring role.

Safety Guidelines and Precautions

Despite Wall Pilates being a low-impact form of exercise, safety is paramount. Always commence your workout sessions with a suitable warm-up to prepare your muscles and joints and conclude with a cool-down phase to aid recovery. Listen to your body's signals and avoid pushing beyond your comfort zone too rapidly – gradual progression is healthier and more sustainable. Pay close attention to your form during each exercise, as improper technique can lead to injuries. Above all, remember that training should be enjoyable, so ensure you're having fun with your Wall Pilates journey.

Now, you are fully prepared to set up a dedicated and safe space for your Wall Pilates practice. Remember, this is a journey of wellness, not a sprint for quick fixes. Every small step is a milestone to enhanced fitness and improved overall health. In the next chapter, we'll guide you on smoothly transitioning into performing Wall Pilates exercises. With your dedication and persistence, every wall in your home holds the potential to become a powerful ally in your health and wellness quest. Let's move forward to the next phase of your Wall Pilates adventure!

Chapter 4: Transitioning to Wall Pilates Exercises

Now that you've cultivated an ideal environment for Wall Pilates in Chapter 3, it's time to enter the practice arena. This chapter is designed to guide you seamlessly into the world of Wall Pilates exercises, addressing all necessary steps and considerations. Here, we'll establish realistic goals, underline the importance of proper form and technique, encourage mindfulness, introduce warm-up and cool-down routines suitable for practitioners of all levels, and provide motivational tips to keep your spirits soaring on this transformative journey.

Setting Realistic Expectations

Your Wall Pilates journey starts with setting attainable, realistic goals. Understand that every person's journey is different, influenced by factors like initial fitness levels, body type, age, and prior experience with Pilates or similar exercises. It's perfectly normal if you can't master all exercises right away. Wall Pilates is about progress, not perfection. So, celebrate each small advancement, and remember to be patient and compassionate with your body. Progress might seem slow initially, but consistency will inevitably lead to improvement.

Importance of Proper Form and Technique

Wall Pilates focuses heavily on form and technique. The correct form ensures that the targeted muscles are engaged and that the risk of injury is minimized. Always engage your core, maintain spinal alignment, and coordinate your movements with your breath. Take the time to understand and perform each exercise accurately, without rushing. This is not a competition; it's a journey of self-discovery and improvement.

The Power of Mindful Practice

One of the cornerstones of Wall Pilates is its emphasis on mindfulness. Each exercise invites you to be wholly present, focusing on your breath, the form, and the movement itself. By clearing your mind of distractions, you cultivate a deeper, more intimate connection with your body. This practice not only enhances your physical performance but also promotes mental clarity, stress reduction, and overall well-being.

Motivation for Success

Beginning a new fitness routine, like Wall Pilates, can feel challenging. Some days, you might struggle to find motivation. During these times, remind yourself of why you started. Each step you take, no matter how tiny, leads you forward on your wellness journey. Consistency is the golden key in fitness. Even if you manage just a few minutes each day, that's still progress. Keep moving, remain dedicated, and the fruits of your efforts will start to manifest.

Armed with these insights, you're fully prepared to step into your Wall Pilates practice. Envision yourself in the personalized space you've created, growing stronger, more flexible, and deeply in tune with your body with each session. Remember, your greatest motivator is you. Believe in your potential and persist in your efforts. As we embark on this journey together, get ready to unlock a new level of fitness and well-being with Wall Pilates.

Chapter 5: Warming Up and Cooling Down for Wall Pilates

Having decided to embark on your Wall Pilates adventure, your eagerness to jump into the core exercises is palpable. Yet, before we unravel the transformative power of Wall Pilates, there's a preparatory step we can't overlook - the warm-up.

This isn't just about ticking off a routine. The warm-up is a cornerstone that guarantees a safe, impactful, and rewarding Wall Pilates experience. Consider it the initial tempo of your fitness symphony. Though the anticipation of exploring Wall Pilates is high, pausing to grasp the essence of a thorough warm-up is paramount.

This section accentuates the warm-up's value before plunging into Wall Pilates. We'll chart a course on priming your body for the exercises ahead, weaving through the best strategies and pro tips. We'll light up every muscle group in preparation, from your head to your toes.

Each second dedicated to warming up enhances the efficacy of the impending workout. Stay patient - those Wall Pilates moves are within reach. Let's lay the groundwork for an exceptional Wall Pilates session. Remember, a compelling overture precedes every grand act. Ready to set things in motion?

How to Warm Up for Wall Pilates

The ideal warm-up encompasses activities that engage all primary muscle groups and echo the patterns you'll soon adopt in your main workout. In Wall Pilates, the warm-up emphasizes flexibility, equilibrium, and mind-body synergy.

Upper Body Warm-up Exercises

Neck Circles

1. Sit or stand upright, shoulders relaxed.
2. Gently lower your chin to your chest.
3. Roll your head to the right, bringing your ear toward the shoulder.

4. Tilt your head back, lifting your chin.

5. Roll your head to the left, bringing your ear toward the shoulder.

6. Bring your chin back to your chest.

Arm Circles

1. With feet shoulder-width apart, stretch your arms out laterally.

2. Initiate small arm circles, gradually enlarging their diameter.

3. After a set, reverse the circle direction.

Core and Lower Body Warm-up Exercises

Hip Circles

1. Maintain an upright posture with feet hip-width apart.

2. With your hands on your waist, move your hips around in a circular motion.

3. After a few, switch the direction.

Leg Swings

1. Stand erect adjacent to a wall, using it for balance if needed.

2. Control the swinging motion of one leg, alternating between forward and backward swings.

3. Swap legs after a set.

Warm-up Best Practices

- Dedicate 10-15 minutes for the warm-up preceding your Wall Pilates routine.

- Prioritize dynamic movements over static stretches to prep your body adequately.

- Be attuned to your body's cues; let your warm-up's vigor reflect your fitness level.

Expert Tips

- The warm-up isn't about depleting energy but readying your physique.

- Uphold an impeccable posture, ensuring effective muscle engagement.

- Breathing is key. Oxygenate your muscles adequately to amplify your warm-up potency.

Embracing the Cool-Down

You've conquered your Wall Pilates session, and you're buzzing with energy. Before you continue your day, let's dedicate five minutes – just a short pause – to transition your body from vigorous activity back to its normal state. This phase called the cool-down, is vital.

Why is it so? The cool-down bridges your intensive workout and regular activity, reducing muscle tension, gradually decreasing your heart rate, and minimizing post-exercise stiffness. It's not uncommon to feel a sensation of muscle soreness or tightness, often referred to as Delayed Onset Muscle Soreness (DOMS). This sensation arises due to the tiny tears that naturally occur in muscle fibers during exercise, which are essential to muscle growth and strengthening. It's perfectly okay to feel this soreness – it's a sign that you've effectively engaged and challenged your muscles.

The cool-down is essential to fully wrap up your Wall Pilates session on a positive note. This section will guide you through a concise yet practical 5-minute cool-down, focusing on stretches that help relax the muscles you've worked on. The cool-down is the perfect moment to reflect on your Wall Pilates achievements and transition smoothly back to your routine.

5-Minute Cool Down After Wall Pilates

Neck Relaxer (20 seconds)

1. Sit comfortably.
2. Gently tilt your head towards one shoulder, holding for 10 seconds.
3. Repeat on the opposite side.

Arm and Shoulder Stretch (40 seconds)

1. Extend one arm straight across your chest.
2. Use the opposite hand to pull the arm closer, stretching the shoulder gently.
3. Hold for 20 seconds, then switch arms.

Hip Flexor Stretch (40 seconds)

1. Start in a lunge position, with one foot forward, and one stretched behind.
2. Gently push your hips forward, feeling a stretch along the front of your back leg's hip.

3. Hold for 20 seconds, then switch legs.

Hamstring Stretch (40 seconds)

1. Sit with one leg extended and the other bent.
2. Reach forward towards your extended foot.
3. Hold for 20 seconds, then switch legs.

Deep Breathing (1 minute)

1. Take deep inhales and exhales to relax your body and mind, facilitating recovery.

Final Thoughts

- This 5-minute cool-down is an essential transition phase post-exercise.
- Maintain deep, controlled breaths throughout to aid relaxation.
- Reflect on your progress and savor the benefits of your Wall Pilates session.

Remember, every Wall Pilates session consists of a warm-up, the main exercises, and concludes with a cool-down. Each phase is pivotal. After cooling down, step forth with pride, feeling refreshed and accomplished.

Chapter 6: Exercises

Congratulations! You've laid the groundwork and warmed up your body. Now you're ready for the moment you've been anticipating – the beginning of your Wall Pilates exercises.

In the coming chapters, you will discover a collection of Wall Pilates exercises I've selected based on their effectiveness and alignment with Wall Pilates principles. Each activity is accompanied by a detailed instructions to ensure you understand each movement and can perform it safely and effectively.

Beyond Traditional Exercise Organization: The Holistic Approach of Wall Pilates

These exercises aren't organized by target muscle. Wall Pilates is a holistic practice engaging several muscles simultaneously. This approach not only builds strength but ensures a balanced development. By not grouping exercises by specific muscles, I encourage a comprehensive view of body conditioning, emphasizing the interconnectedness of our forces. While you'll have insights on the primary muscles each exercise impacts, remember that Wall Pilates is about the bigger picture of overall strength, balance, and well-being.

Back to the exercises, I encourage you to explore and experiment. Some activities will resonate more with you, while others might challenge you. It's all part of the journey. Pilates is about patience, precision, and mindfulness. Discover what works best for you at your own pace.

After mastering the individual exercises, there's a 28-day challenge to help you initiate and maintain your practice, providing structure if you need help determining where to begin.

Remember, your Wall Pilates journey is personal. Each exercise is a step towards a healthier, fitter you. While you might be eager to start training, I've included bonus chapters. It can enrich your experience, and I recommend reading it before diving into the exercises. Trust me. It's worth the page-turn. **Pages: 92, 96**.

Wall Plank

• Target Muscle: Core muscles (transversus abdominis, rectus abdominis, and obliques), shoulder stabilizers.

• Who Can Do It: Suitable for ranging from beginners to advanced. It's also an excellent option for seniors and those recovering from injuries, offering a lower-impact way to strengthen the core. Always consult with a healthcare professional before beginning any new exercise.

• Benefits: The Wall Plank strengthens your core and shoulder stabilizers, which can improve posture, reduce lower back pain, and increase functional strength for daily activities. It also encourages better balance and stability.

• Form and Alignment Tips: Maintain a straight line from your head to your heels. Ensure your shoulders are stacked directly above your wrists. Activate your core muscles and tighten your glutes to maintain a stable body position.

• Breathing: Inhale at the starting position. Exhale as you move into the plank. Inhale while holding the plank. Exhale as you return to the starting position.

• Modification: Keep your feet closer to the wall to modify.

• Safety Precautions: Make sure you have a sturdy wall with enough space around you. If you feel discomfort in your wrists or shoulders, adjust your hand position or take a break.

• Repetition and Sets: Start with holding the plank for 20 seconds. Gradually build up to 1 minute. Perform 2-3 sets.

• Rest Period: Rest for 30 seconds to 1 minute between sets.

• Notes: If you feel pain in your lower back, it may indicate that you're not correctly engaging your core. Take a moment to reset and ensure the proper form.

Instructions:

1. Assume a standing position facing a wall with your feet hip-width apart.

2. Ensure your palms are placed firmly against the wall, shoulder-width apart, with your arms bent.

3. Walk your feet back as you lean forward until you're in a diagonal plank position.

4. Hold this position, keeping your body straight and your abs engaged.

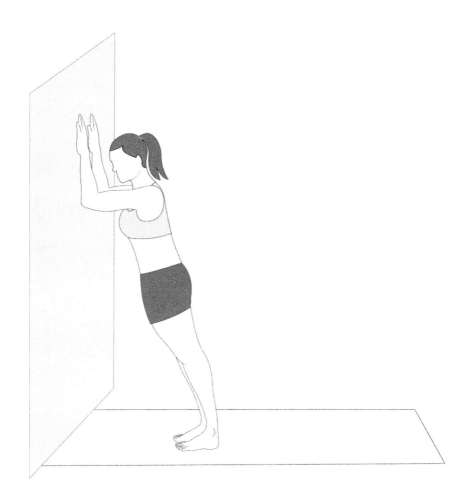

Wall-Assisted Bridge

• Target Muscle: Glutes, Hamstrings, Lower Back.

• Who Can Do It: Ideal for all fitness levels, seniors, and those recovering from lower body injuries. Consult a healthcare professional before starting new exercises.

• Benefits: Strengthens and tones the glutes and hamstrings, stretches the hip flexors, and enhances core stability and posture.

• Form and Alignment Tips: Keep feet flat and hip-width apart. Your hips should lift just a bit above the floor.

• Common Mistakes to Avoid: Don't let your knees cave in or push your hips too high.

• Breathing: Inhale when you lower your hips; exhale as you lift.

• Modification and Progression: Lift hips less high for modification. For progression, try one-legged bridges.

• Safety Precautions: Ensure sturdy footing against the wall and avoid straining your neck.

• Repetition and Sets: Start with 10-15 reps for 2-3 sets.

• Rest Period: Rest for 30 seconds to 1 minute between sets.

• Notes: Focus on activating your glute muscles throughout the lift rather than solely relying on your lower back.

Instructions:

1. Start by lying down on your back. Ensure your knees are bent, creating a comfortably wide angle, and place your feet flat against the wall.

2. Push your feet into the wall and gently lift your hips above the ground.

3. Lower your hips back down to the starting position. Repeat.

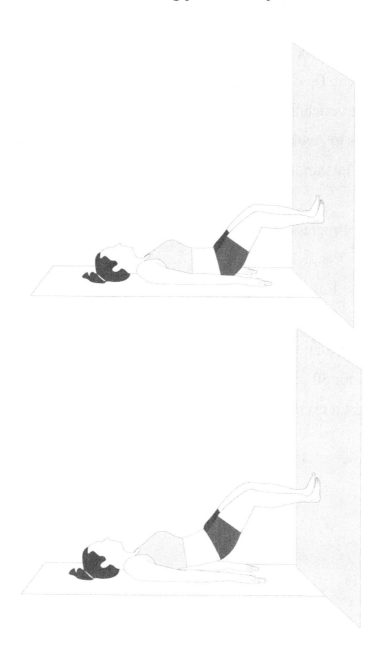

Wall Roll-Down

• Target Muscle: Spinal muscles, Hamstrings, Glutes.

• Who Can Do It: This is beneficial for everyone, including beginners, seniors, and those recovering from injuries. As always, consult a healthcare professional before starting new exercises.

• Benefits: It promotes spinal mobility, stretches and strengthens the back and hamstring muscles, and helps in enhancing posture.

• Form and Alignment Tips: Maintain a soft bend in your knees, keep your spine long, and roll down and down one vertebra at a time.

• Common Mistakes to Avoid: Avoid locking your knees and rounding your shoulders.

• Breathing: Inhale to start. Exhale as you roll down. Inhale at the bottom. Exhale as you roll back up.

• Modification and Progression: To modify, don't bend as far. To progress, increase the range of motion.

• Safety Precautions: Ensure a flat and sturdy wall. Avoid this exercise if you have severe lower back problems.

• Repetition and Sets: Start with 8-10 reps for 2-3 sets.

• Rest Period: Rest for 30 seconds to 1 minute between sets.

• Notes: This is a great exercise to improve flexibility and relieve tension in the back.

Instructions:

1. Stand with your back to the wall and feet hip-width apart.

2. Extend your arms down alongside your body.

3. Inhale to prepare. As you exhale, tuck your chin into your chest and roll down and away from the wall, one vertebra at a time.

4. Hang at the bottom of your roll-down with your hands hanging towards the floor.

5. Inhale at the bottom, then exhale as you roll back up to the starting position, pressing your back into the wall.

6. Repeat this movement with smooth, controlled motion.

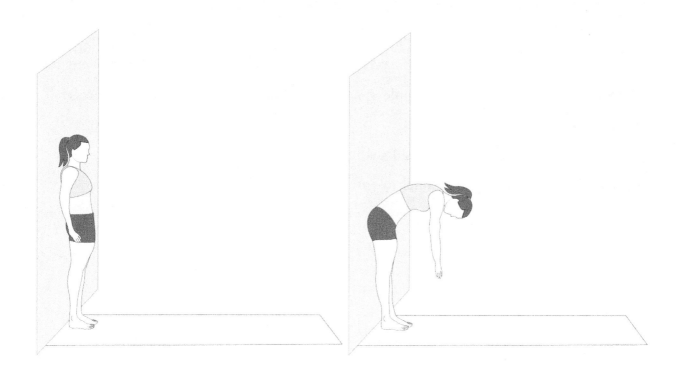

Wall-Assisted Knees Side to Side

• Target Muscle: Obliques, Hip Flexors, Lower Back.

• Who Can Do It: Suitable for all fitness levels, seniors, and those recovering from injuries. Consult a healthcare professional before starting new exercises.

• Benefits: Increases hip mobility, strengthens the core, and helps improve balance and stability.

• Form and Alignment Tips: Keep your back flat on the floor and maintain control as you move your legs from side to side.

• Common Mistakes to Avoid: Avoid lifting your back off the floor and moving your legs too quickly.

• Breathing: Inhale as you move your knees to one side; exhale as you return them to the center.

• Modification and Progression: To progress, straighten your legs or add ankle weights.

• Safety Precautions: Ensure ample space and a sturdy wall. Avoid this exercise if you have hip issues.

• Repetition and Sets: Start with 20 swings (10 on each side) for 2-3 sets.

• Rest Period: Rest for 30 seconds to 1 minute between sets.

• Notes: This exercise is excellent for increasing mobility and flexibility in the lower body.

Instructions:

1. Start by lying on your back with your head away from the wall and your legs bent up on the wall.

2. Place your arms out to your sides for support.

3. Keeping your back flat on the floor, slowly swing your knees from side to side, moving as a unit.

4. Control the movement and return your knees to the center before swinging to the other side.

5. That's one repetition. Continue to repeat this movement.

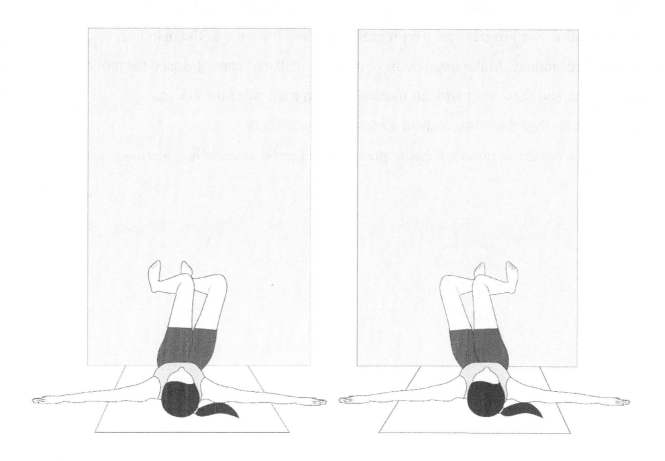

Wall Marches

• Target Muscle: Hip Flexors, Core, Quads.

• Who Can Do It: Suitable for all fitness levels, seniors, and those with balance issues. Always consult with a healthcare professional before starting new exercises.

• Benefits: Enhances balance, strengthens the lower body, and improves coordination.

• Form and Alignment Tips: Stand tall, keep your core engaged, and lift your knees high with each march.

• Common Mistakes to Avoid: Don't round your back or let your arms droop down.

• Breathing: Inhale as you lift one knee, exhale as you lower it. Repeat with the other knee.

• Modification and Progression: To progress, increase the pace of the marches.

• Safety Precautions: Make sure you have a sturdy wall and enough space for movement.

• Repetition and Sets: Start with 20 marches (10 on each side) for 2-3 sets.

• Rest Period: Rest for 30 seconds to 1 minute between sets.

• Notes: This exercise promotes better posture and can be an excellent warm-up activity.

Instructions:

1. Stand facing a wall with your feet hip-width apart. Extend your arms straight and place your hands on the wall at shoulder height.

2. Raise your right knee upwards, ensuring your back remains straight and your hands stay pressed against the wall.

3. Lower your right foot back to the floor.

4. Now, repeat the same motion with your left knee.

5. Continue to march in place, alternating knees.

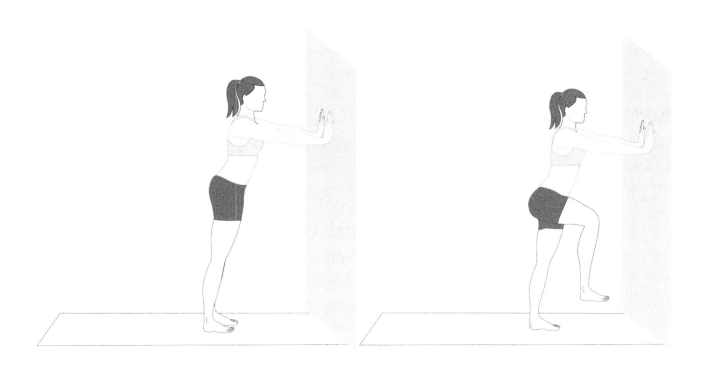

Wall Glute Kickbacks

• Target Muscle: Glutes, Hamstrings.

• Who Can Do It: Suitable for all fitness levels, seniors, and those with balance issues. Always consult with a healthcare professional before starting new exercises.

• Benefits: Strengthens and tones the glutes and hamstrings, enhances hip mobility, improves core stability, and contributes to better balance.

• Form and Alignment Tips: Keep a slight bend in your arms, extend your leg straight back from the hip while maintaining a straight spine, and ensure you're squeezing your glutes at the top of each kickback.

• Common Mistakes to Avoid: Avoid arching your back and be careful not to hyperextend your knee or swing your leg. The movement should be controlled.

• Breathing: Inhale as you prepare the move; exhale as you kick your leg back; inhale as you return the leg to the starting position.

• Modification and Progression: To modify, perform the kickback with less range of motion. To progress, add ankle weights or increase the speed while maintaining control.

• Safety Precautions: Ensure you have a sturdy wall for support and plenty of space for movement. Be mindful not to strain your neck.

• Repetition and Sets: Start with 10-15 kickbacks on each leg for 2-3 sets.

• Rest Period: Rest for 30 seconds to 1 minute between sets.

• Notes: Focus on the quality of movement rather than the quantity of repetitions. It's about engaging and activating the glutes effectively.

Instructions:

1. Stand facing a wall with your feet hip-width apart. Place your hands on the wall, keeping a slight bend in your arms.

2. Engage your core and extend your right leg straight behind you, while keeping your toes pointed towards the ground.

3. Squeeze your glutes at the top of the movement, then lower your leg back to the starting position in a controlled manner.

4. Repeat the movement on your left leg. Continue to alternate legs for the duration of the set.

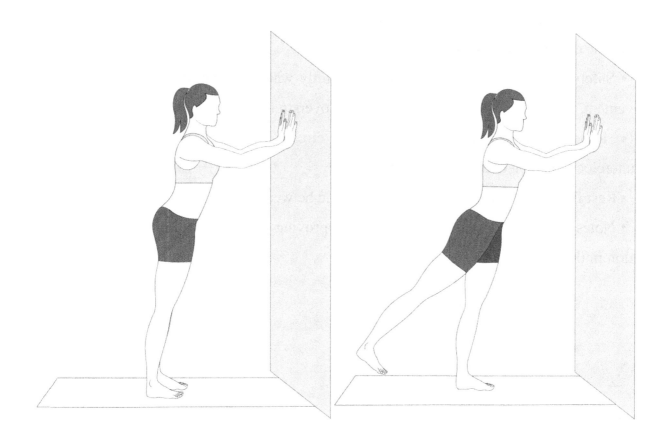

Wall Leg Circles

• Target Muscle: Hip Flexors, Quads, Glutes, Core.

• Who Can Do It: Suitable for all fitness levels, seniors, and those with balance issues. As always, consult with a healthcare professional before starting new exercises.

• Benefits: Increases hip mobility, strengthens and tones the lower body, enhances core stability and improves balance.

• Form and Alignment Tips: Lean slightly into the wall, keep your core engaged, and ensure you're making controlled, smooth circles with your legs.

• Common Mistakes to Avoid: Avoid fast, jerky movements or swinging the leg too wildly. Also, ensure your standing leg remains stable.

• Breathing: Inhale as you start the circle, exhale as you complete it.

• Modification and Progression: To modify, make smaller circles. To progress, increase the size of the circles or add ankle weights.

• Safety Precautions: Ensure you have a sturdy wall for support and plenty of space for movement. Be careful not to strain your neck or overstretch your leg.

• Repetition and Sets: Start with 15 circles in each direction (clockwise and counterclockwise) on each leg for 2-3 sets.

• Rest Period: Rest for 30 seconds to 1 minute between sets.

• Notes: This is an excellent exercise for improving flexibility and increasing the range of motion in the hips.

Instructions:

1. Stand with your back to a wall with your feet hip-width apart. Lean slightly into the wall for support.

2. Lift your right leg and draw a circle with your foot, keeping your toes pointed and your leg straight.

3. Complete the circle and then reverse the direction, drawing a circle in the opposite direction.

4. Lower your right leg and repeat the same sequence with your left leg.

5. Continue to alternate legs for the duration of the set. Remember, control is vital in this exercise.

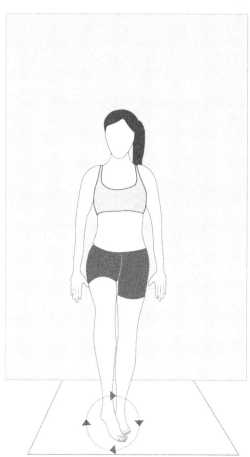

Wall Calf Raises

- Target Muscle: Calves (Gastrocnemius and Soleus).

- Who Can Do It: Suitable for all fitness levels, seniors, and those with balance issues. As always, consult with a healthcare professional before starting new exercises.

- Benefits: Strengthens and tones the calves, improves balance, and enhances ankle stability.

- Form and Alignment Tips: Stand tall, keep your core engaged, and ensure you lift from your heels, not your toes.

- Common Mistakes to Avoid: Don't round your back or let your heels touch the floor between repetitions.

- Breathing: Inhale as you lower your heels, exhale as you lift them.

- Modification and Progression: Add repetitions or hold at the top of the lift for a couple of seconds to progress.

- Safety Precautions: Ensure you have a sturdy wall for support. Be mindful not to strain your neck.

- Repetition and Sets: Start with 15-20 raises for 2-3 sets.

- Rest Period: Rest for 30 seconds to 1 minute between sets.

- Notes: This exercise can be performed at any point during your workout, but it's especially beneficial as a warm-up or cool-down exercise.

Instructions:

1. Stand facing a wall with your feet hip-width apart and your hands on the wall for support.

2. Elevate your heels, rising onto your toes as high as possible.

3. Slowly lower your heels back to the ground.

4. Repeat the movement for the duration of the set, keeping your movements smooth and controlled.

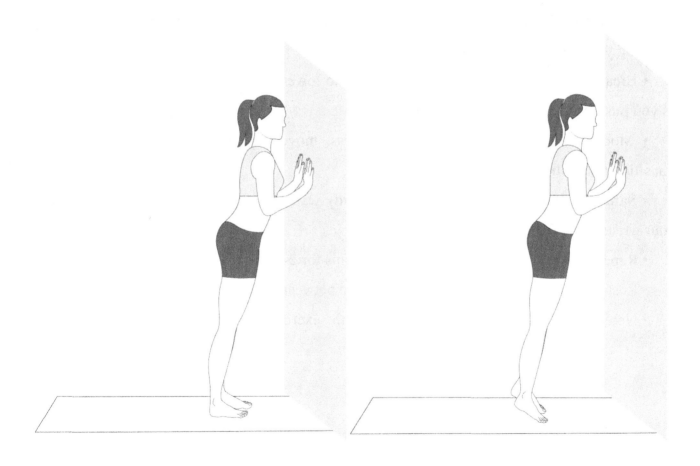

Wall Push-Ups

• Target Muscle: Chest (Pectorals), Arms (Triceps), Shoulders (Deltoids).

• Who Can Do It: Suitable for all fitness levels, seniors, and those looking for a lower-impact version of traditional push-ups. As always, consult with a healthcare professional before starting new exercises.

• Benefits: Strengthens and tones the upper body, improves functional strength, and enhances shoulder stability.

• Form and Alignment Tips: Keep your body in a straight line from head to heels. Ensure your hands are shoulder-width apart and your elbows are close to your body.

• Common Mistakes to Avoid: Avoid sagging your hips, flaring your elbows out wide, or straining your neck by looking up or down.

• Breathing: Inhale as you bend your elbows to lower your chest towards the wall, exhale as you push back to the starting position.

• Modification and Progression: To progress, move your feet away from the wall or transition to traditional push-ups when ready.

• Safety Precautions: Ensure you have a sturdy wall for support. Be mindful not to strain your wrists.

• Repetition and Sets: Start with 10-15 push-ups for 2-3 sets.

• Rest Period: Rest for 30 seconds to 1 minute between sets.

• Notes: Keep your core engaged throughout the exercise to help maintain proper form.

Instructions:

1. Stand facing a wall with your feet hip-width apart. Place your hands on the wall at shoulder height and shoulder width apart.

2. Step back until your arms are fully extended, but keep your feet firmly planted.

3. Bend your elbows and lower your chest towards the wall while keeping your body straight.

4. Push yourself back to the starting position once your face almost touches the wall.

5. Repeat the movement for the duration of the set, keeping your movements smooth and controlled.

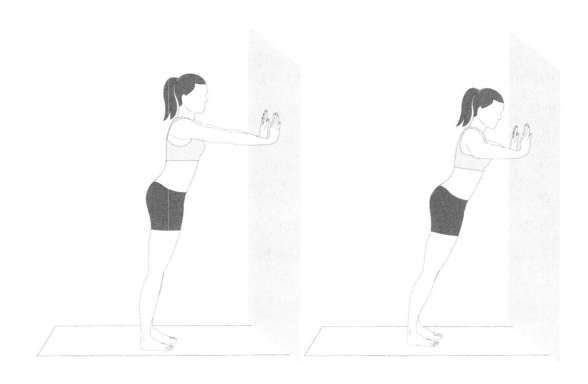

Wall Triceps Dips

• Target Muscle: Triceps, Shoulders (Deltoids).

• Who Can Do It: Suitable for all fitness levels, seniors, and those looking for a lower-impact version of traditional triceps dips. As always, consult with a healthcare professional before starting new exercises.

• Benefits: Strengthens and tones the triceps and shoulders and improves upper body functional strength.

• Form and Alignment Tips: Keep your body close to the wall and your elbows close to your body. Ensure your hands are shoulder-width apart.

• Common Mistakes to Avoid: Avoid flaring your elbows out or straining your neck by looking up or down.

• Breathing: Inhale as you bend your elbows to lower your body towards the wall, exhale as you push back to the starting position.

• Modification and Progression: To progress, move your feet away from the wall or transition to traditional triceps dips when ready.

• Safety Precautions: Ensure you have a sturdy wall for support. Be mindful not to strain your wrists.

• Repetition and Sets: Start with 10-15 dips for 2-3 sets.

• Rest Period: Rest for 30 seconds to 1 minute between sets.

• Notes: Keep your core engaged throughout the exercise to help maintain proper form.

Instructions:

1. Stand facing the wall with your feet hip-width apart.

2. While keeping your body straight, place your forearms on the wall, with your elbows bent. Ensure that your elbows are pointing directly downward towards the floor rather than flaring out to the sides. Fingers should point upwards.

3. Lower your body towards the wall until your face almost touches it.

4. Push yourself back to the starting position by fully extending your arms.

5. Ensure your movements are smooth and controlled, and repeat for the desired number of repetitions.

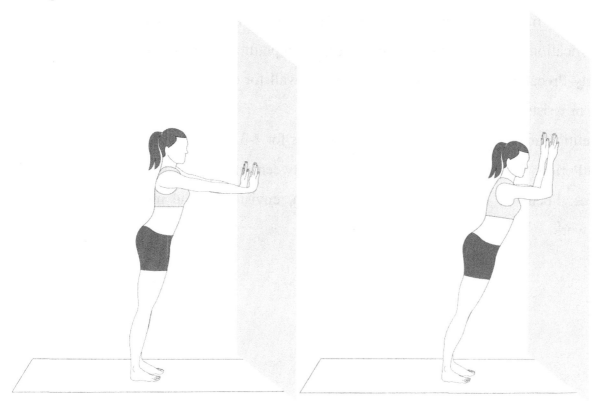

Wall Lateral Pull Downs

• Target Muscle: Upper Back (Latissimus Dorsi), Shoulders (Deltoids).

• Who Can Do It: Suitable for all fitness levels, seniors, and those seeking a low-impact upper body exercise. As always, consult with a healthcare professional before starting new exercises.

• Benefits: Strengthens and tones the upper back and shoulders, improves posture and upper body functional strength.

• Common Mistakes to Avoid: Avoid rounding your back, shrugging your shoulders, or pulling with your hands instead of your back muscles.

• Breathing: Inhale as you extend your arms upwards, exhale as you pull down.

• Modification and Progression: To progress, add repetitions or increase the pull speed.

• Safety Precautions: Ensure you have a sturdy wall for support. Be mindful not to strain your neck or wrists.

• Repetition and Sets: Start with 10-15 pull downs for 2-3 sets.

• Rest Period: Rest for 30 seconds to 1 minute between sets.

• Notes: Focus on the mind-muscle connection, envisioning the muscles in your back doing the work.

Instructions:

1. Stand with your back to a wall, feet hip-width apart and slightly away from the wall.

2. Extend your arms upwards and place backs of your hands on the wall behind you, shoulder-width apart.

3. Keeping your core tight, pull your elbows down, squeezing your shoulder blades together.

4. Extend your arms, reaching the wall to complete the movement.

5. Repeat for the recommended number of repetitions, keeping the motion controlled and smooth.

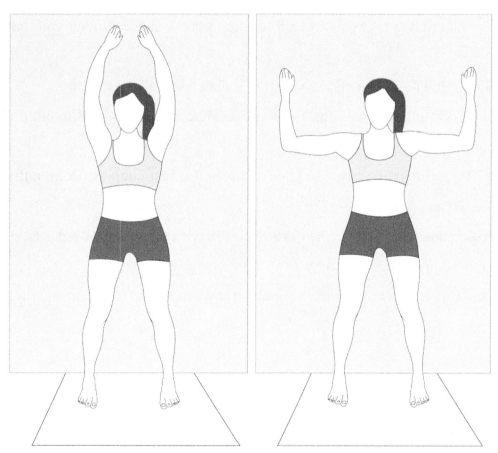

Wall Arm Circles

• Target Muscle: Shoulders (Deltoids), Upper Back.

• Who Can Do It: Suitable for everyone, seniors and those seeking a low-impact upper body exercise. As always, consult with a healthcare professional before starting new exercises.

• Benefits: Increases shoulder mobility and strength and promotes better posture.

• Form and Alignment Tips: Stand tall with your back flat against the wall, arms straight down. Raise your arms to the sides and over your head, then lower them down again in a controlled, circular motion.

• Common Mistakes to Avoid: Avoid bending your arms or arching your back away from the wall.

• Breathing: Inhale as you raise your arms, exhale as you lower them.

• Modification and Progression: To progress, increase the range of motion or the speed of the circles.

• Safety Precautions: Ensure you have a sturdy wall for support. Be mindful not to strain your neck or wrists.

• Repetition and Sets: Start with 10-15 circles in each direction for 2-3 sets.

• Rest Period: Rest for 30 seconds to 1 minute between sets.

• Notes: Keep your core engaged throughout the exercise to maintain stability.

Instructions:

1. Stand with your back pressed firmly against a wall. Your feet should be about hip-width apart.
2. Extend your arms straight down at your sides, with the backs of your hands touching the wall.
3. Slowly raise your arms, keeping the back of your hands and arms in contact with the wall.
4. Continue to raise your arms, tracing a circle along the wall until they reach overhead. At the topmost position, the backs of your hands should still be in contact with the wall.
5. Slowly lower them back down in a circular motion to the starting position.
6. Keep your movements smooth and controlled. You can reverse the direction of the circles after a set number of repetitions for balanced training.
7. Perform the movement for the desired number of repetitions.

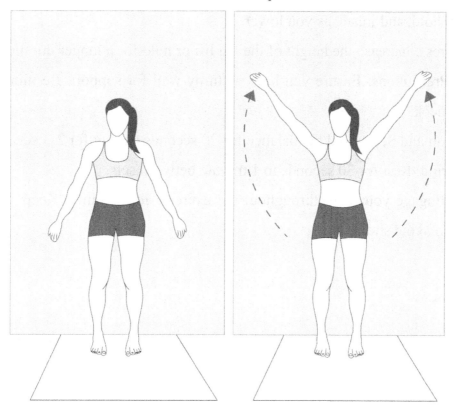

Single Leg Balance

• Target Muscle: Core, Glutes, and Hamstrings.

• Who Can Do It: Suitable for everyone, especially beginners, seniors, and those recovering from leg, ankle, or balance issues. Always consult with a healthcare professional before starting new exercises.

• Benefits: Enhances balance, strengthens the core, and tones the glutes and hamstrings.

• Form and Alignment Tips: Stand facing the wall, lean slightly into the wall with one hand for support. Lift one leg off the ground and hold it slightly back. Maintain a straight line from your head to your lifted foot.

• Common Mistakes to Avoid: Avoid leaning too much into the wall or letting your hip open out to the side.

• Breathing: Maintain a steady breathing pattern throughout. Inhale as you lift your leg, exhale as you hold, and inhale as you lower.

• To progress, increase the height of the leg lift or hold for a longer duration.

• Safety Precautions: Ensure you have a sturdy wall for support. Be mindful not to strain your wrist or neck.

• Repetition and Sets: Hold the balance for 20 seconds per leg for 2-3 sets.

• Rest Period: Rest for 30 seconds to 1 minute between sets.

• Notes: Engage your core throughout the exercise for stability. Keep the standing knee slightly bent to avoid strain.

Instructions:

1. Stand facing the wall, a few feet away.

2. Extend one hand to touch the wall for balance lightly.

3. Shift your weight onto one foot and slowly lift the other foot off the ground, extending it slightly back.

4. Hold the balance for the recommended duration, keeping your gaze fixed at a point for focus.

5. Lower your foot back to the ground in a controlled manner, then repeat the exercise on the other side.

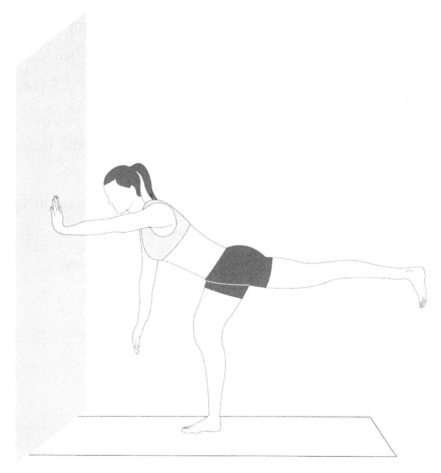

Wall Mountain Climbers

• Target Muscle: Core (especially lower abs), Quads, and Shoulders.

• Who Can Do It: Suitable for beginners and advanced fitness enthusiasts. Also suitable for seniors and those with balance issues. Always consult a healthcare professional before starting new exercises.

• Benefits: Strengthens and tones the core, improves cardiovascular endurance, and enhances balance and coordination.

• Form and Alignment Tips: Stand facing the wall with your hands placed flat against it. Quickly alternate, like running in place, bringing each knee towards your chest.

• Common Mistakes to Avoid: Avoid bending your back or hunching your shoulders.

• Breathing: Inhale as you bring one knee up, exhale as you switch legs.

• Modification and Progression: To modify, slow down the pace. Increase the speed or add a small jump as you switch legs to progress.

• Safety Precautions: Ensure you have a sturdy wall for support. Be mindful not to strain your wrists or shoulders.

• Repetition and Sets: Start with 20-30 seconds of continuous movement for 2-3 sets.

• Rest Period: Rest for 30 seconds to 1 minute between sets.

• Notes: Keep your core engaged and your movements controlled.

Instructions:

1. Stand facing the wall and place your hands flat against it at shoulder height and slightly wider than shoulder-width apart.

2. Start with your feet hip-width apart.

3. Quickly bring one knee to your chest, then return it to the ground. Immediately repeat with the other leg.

4. Continue alternating legs, similar to running in place, for the recommended duration.

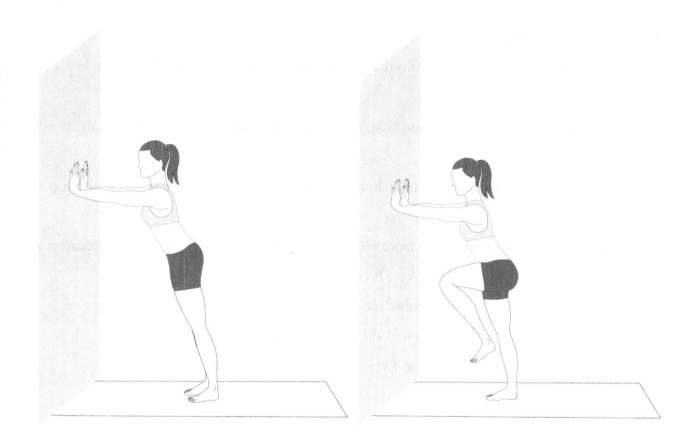

Wall Bridge

• Target Muscle: Glutes, Hamstrings, and Lower Back.

• Who Can Do It: Suitable for beginners, seniors, and those recovering from lower body or back injuries. Always consult with a healthcare professional before starting new exercises.

• Benefits: Strengthens the glutes and hamstrings, enhances lower back strength and flexibility, and improves hip mobility.

• Form and Alignment Tips: Start lying on your back with your knees bent and feet flat on the wall. Press down through your heels and lift your hips off the floor until your thighs and torso form a straight line.

• Common Mistakes to Avoid: Avoid hyperextending your back or lifting your heels off the wall.

• Breathing: Inhale as you lift your hips, exhale as you hold the bridge, and inhale as you lower.

• Progression: Hold the bridge for a longer duration or add a small pulse at the top to progress.

• Safety Precautions: Ensure you have a sturdy wall for support. If you feel discomfort in your lower back, lower your hips or take a break.

• Repetition and Sets: Hold the bridge for 20 seconds for 2-3 sets.

• Rest Period: Rest for 30 seconds to 1 minute between sets.

• Notes: Keep your core engaged and your movements controlled.

Instructions:

1. Start by lying on your back, feet flat on the wall, knees bent, forming a comfortably wide angle.

2. Place your arms flat on the ground by your sides.

3. Push through your heels and lift your hips off the ground, creating a straight line from your knees to your shoulders.

4. Hold the position for the recommended duration.

5. Lower your hips back to the ground in a controlled manner, then repeat.

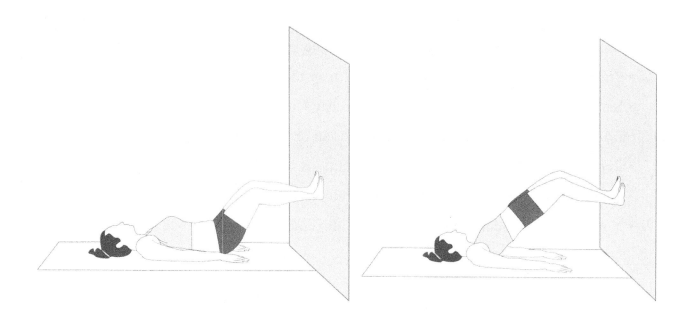

Wall Scissor Kicks

• Target Muscle: Lower Abs, Inner and Outer Thighs.

• Who Can Do It: Suitable for everyone, especially beginners, seniors, and those recovering from lower body or core injuries. Always consult with a healthcare professional before starting new exercises.

• Benefits: Strengthens the lower abs and tones the inner and outer thighs. Enhances lower body flexibility and hip mobility.

• Form and Alignment Tips: Start lying on your back with your legs straight up against the wall. Keeping your legs straight, open them out to the sides like a pair of scissors and then bring them back together.

• Common Mistakes to Avoid: Avoid bending your knees or lifting your lower back off the floor.

• Breathing: Inhale as you open your legs, exhale, and bring them back together.

• Progression: To progress, add ankle weights or increase the speed of the movement.

• Safety Precautions: Ensure you have a sturdy wall for support. If you feel discomfort in your hips or lower back, reduce the range of motion or take a break.

• Repetition and Sets: Start with 12-15 repetitions for 2-3 sets.

• Rest Period: Rest for 30 seconds to 1 minute between sets.

• Notes: Keep your core engaged and your movements controlled.

Instructions:

1. Start by lying on your back with your legs straight up against the wall, feet together.

2. Keeping your legs straight, open them out to the sides like a pair of scissors.

3. Slowly bring your legs back together with control.

4. Repeat for the recommended number of repetitions.

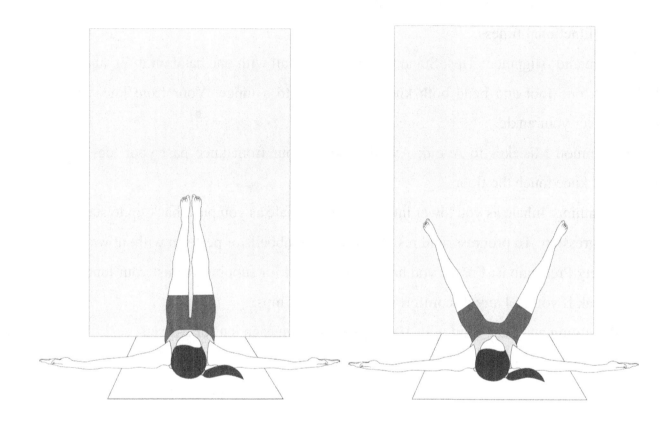

Wall-Assisted Lunges

• Target Muscle: Glutes, Quadriceps, and Hamstrings.

• Who Can Do It: Suitable for everyone, from beginners to advanced. Particularly beneficial for seniors or those needing additional balance support. Always consult with a healthcare professional before starting new exercises.

• Benefits: Strengthens the lower body muscles, improves balance and coordination, and enhances functional fitness.

• Form and Alignment Tips: Stand parallel to the wall with one hand on it for support. Step back with one foot and bend both knees to lower into a lunge. Your front knee should be directly over your ankle.

• Common Mistakes to Avoid: Avoid bending your front knee past your toes or letting your back knee touch the floor.

• Breathing: Inhale as you lower into the lunge, exhale as you push back up to standing.

• Progression: To progress, add resistance with dumbbells or perform without wall support.

• Safety Precautions: Ensure you have a sturdy wall for support. Adjust your lunge form or take a break if you feel any discomfort in your knees or hips.

• Repetition and Sets: Start with 10-12 repetitions on each leg for 2-3 sets.

• Rest Period: Rest for 30 seconds to 1 minute between sets.

• Notes: Keep your core engaged and maintain an upright posture throughout the exercise.

Instructions:

1. Stand parallel to the wall, about an arm's length away, and place one hand on it for support.

2. Step back with one foot, keeping both feet hip-width apart.

3. Bend both knees to lower into a lunge, keeping your front knee directly over your ankle.

4. Push through your front heel to return to standing, keeping your hand on the wall for balance.

5. Repeat for the recommended number of repetitions, then switch sides.

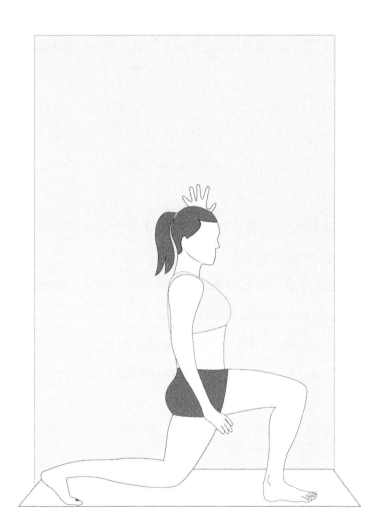

Wall Single Leg Bridge

- Target Muscle: Glutes, Hamstrings, and Core.

- Who Can Do It: Suitable for everyone from beginners to advanced. Particularly beneficial for those looking to enhance lower body strength and stability. Always consult with a healthcare professional before starting new exercises.

- Benefits: Strengthens glutes, hamstrings, and core. It enhances hip mobility and stability and improves balance.

- Form and Alignment Tips: Start lying on your back with one foot on the wall, knee bent at a 90-degree angle. Lift your other leg straight up. Push through the heel on the wall to lift your hips.

- Common Mistakes to Avoid: Avoid lifting your hips too high or letting your lower back arch excessively.

- Breathing: Inhale as you lift your hips, exhale as you hold the bridge, and inhale as you lower.

- Modification and Progression: To modify, keep both feet on the wall. To progress, add a leg extension at the top of the bridge.

- Safety Precautions: Ensure you have a sturdy wall for support. If you feel discomfort in your lower back, lower your hips or take a break.

- Repetition and Sets: Start with 10-12 repetitions on each leg for 2-3 sets.

- Rest Period: Rest for 30 seconds to 1 minute between sets.

- Notes: Keep your core engaged and your movements controlled.

Instructions:

1. Start by lying on your back, one foot on the wall, and your knee bent at a 90-degree angle. The second leg is bent at the knee and raised up.

2. Push through the heel on the wall and lift your hips off the ground, keeping your other leg elevated.

3. Hold the position for a moment, then lower your hips back to the ground with control.

4. Repeat for the recommended number of repetitions, then switch legs.

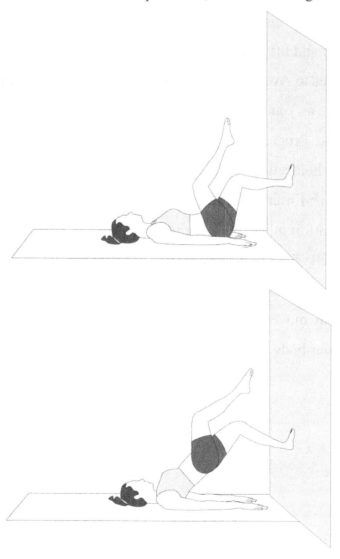

Wall Abdominal Crunches

• Target Muscle: Abdominals.

• Who Can Do It: Suitable for everyone, from beginners to advanced, especially those needing to avoid neck or lower back strain. Always consult with a healthcare professional before starting new exercises.

• Benefits: Strengthens the abdominal muscles, enhances core stability, and can improve posture.

• Form and Alignment Tips: Start lying on your back with your legs straight up against the wall. Engage your core and lift your shoulders off the ground to perform a crunch.

• Common Mistakes to Avoid: Avoid pulling on your neck or rounding your lower back.

• Breathing: Exhale as you lift your upper body. Inhale as you lower.

• Modification and Progression: To modify, bend your knees slightly. Add a twist to engage the obliques or hold a weight to your chest to progress.

• Safety Precautions: Ensure you have a sturdy wall for support. Adjust your form or take a break if you feel discomfort in your neck or lower back.

• Repetition and Sets: Start with 10-15 repetitions for 2-3 sets.

• Rest Period: Rest for 30 seconds to 1 minute between sets.

• Notes: Keep your movements slow and controlled. The focus is on the contraction of your abs, not lifting your body high off the ground.

Instructions:

1. Start by lying on your back with your legs straight up against the wall, feet together.

2. Place your hands behind your head or crossed over your chest.

3. Exhale and engage your core to lift your shoulders off the ground, crunching towards your knees.

4. Inhale and lower back down with control, keeping your legs against the wall.

5. Repeat for the recommended number of repetitions.

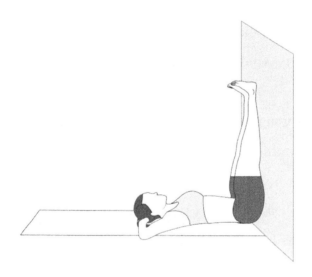

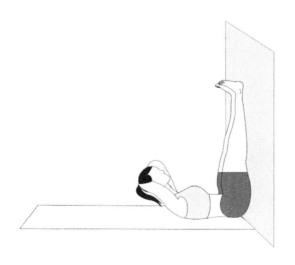

Wall-Assisted Squat (Sliding)

• Target Muscle: Quadriceps, Glutes, and Hamstrings.

• Who Can Do It: Suitable for all levels, especially those needing additional balance support or are new to squats. Always consult with a healthcare professional before starting new exercises.

• Benefits: Strengthens the lower body, improves posture, enhances balance, and aids functional movement.

• Form and Alignment Tips: Stand with your back against the wall. Lower down as if you're sitting back into a chair, then push back up.

• Common Mistakes to Avoid: Avoid letting your knees go past your toes or allowing your lower back to round.

• Breathing: Inhale as you lower the squat, exhale as you push back up.

• Modification and Progression: To modify, don't go as low. To progress, add a resistance band around your thighs or hold weight.

• Safety Precautions: Ensure you have a sturdy wall for support. Adjust your form or take a break if you feel discomfort in your knees or lower back.

• Repetition and Sets: Start with 10-15 repetitions for 2-3 sets.

• Rest Period: Rest for 30 seconds to 1 minute between sets.

• Notes: Engage your core and keep your chest lifted. Focus on pushing through your heels as you rise.

Instructions:

1. Stand with your back against the wall, feet hip-width apart and a step away from the wall.

2. Inhale and lower your body by bending your knees and sliding down the wall until your thighs parallel the floor.

3. Exhale and push through your heels to slide back up the wall to the starting position.

4. Repeat for the recommended number of repetitions.

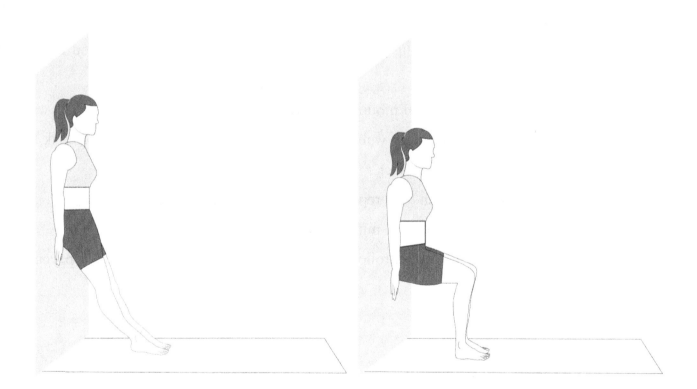

Wall Leg Extension

• Target Muscle: Quadriceps, Glutes, Hamstrings.

• Who Can Do It: Suitable for everyone, especially those looking to strengthen lower body muscles. Consult with a healthcare professional before starting.

• Benefits: Strengthens quadriceps, glutes, and hamstrings, aids in improving balance, and assists in enhancing body coordination.

• Form and Alignment Tips: Start the exercise by placing your knees on the ground at a 90-degree angle, your feet against the wall, your hands flat on the floor, with your body elevated.

• Common Mistakes to Avoid: Avoid arching your back and ensure your neck is relaxed and in line with your spine.

• Breathing: Exhale while extending your legs and lifting your hips. Inhale as you lower back down.

• Modification: Reduce the range of motion for a more accessible.

• Safety Precautions: Ensure a sturdy wall for support. Adjust your form or take a break if discomfort is felt in the knees or lower back.

• Repetition and Sets: Begin with 8-10 repetitions, performing 2-3 sets.

• Rest Period: Rest for 30 seconds to 1 minute between sets.

• Notes: Keep your movements controlled, engage your core throughout, and keep your hands on the floor for balance.

Instructions:

1. Start the exercise by placing your knees on the ground at a 90-degree angle, your feet against the wall, your hands flat on the floor, with your body elevated.

2. Extend your body, lifting your buttocks upwards and straightening your legs so they are no longer at a 90-degree angle.

3. Inhale, slowly lower your hips, and bend your knees, returning to the starting position.

4. Repeat this for the suggested number of repetitions and sets.

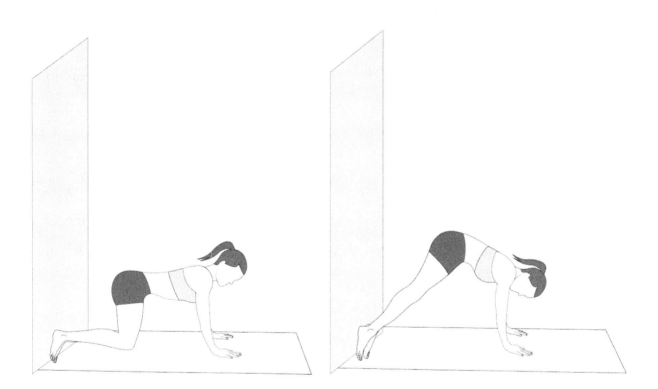

Wall-Assisted Diamond Push-Ups

• Target Muscle: Triceps, Chest (Pectoralis Major), Front Shoulders (Anterior Deltoids).

• Who Can Do It: Suitable for beginners to intermediate fitness enthusiasts. Consult with a healthcare professional before starting a new exercise routine.

• Benefits: Strengthens the triceps, chest, and shoulders. It also enhances upper body strength and stability.

• Form and Alignment Tips: Stand facing the wall and place your hands in a diamond shape on the wall. Keep your body straight as you bend your elbows to lower your body toward the wall.

• Common Mistakes to Avoid: Avoid flaring your elbows out to the sides or letting your hips sag.

• Breathing: Inhale as you lower your body towards the wall, exhale as you push away from the wall.

• Modification and Progression: Move your feet closer to the wall for a more accessible variant. Move your feet away or transition to a floor diamond push-up for more challenges.

• Safety Precautions: Ensure a sturdy wall. Adjust your form or take a break if you feel discomfort in your wrists or shoulders.

• Repetition and Sets: Begin with 8-10 repetitions, performing 2-3 sets.

• Rest Period: Rest for 30 seconds to 1 minute between sets.

• Notes: Remember to engage your core to help maintain a straight body line.

Instructions:

1. Stand facing the wall and place your hands on the wall in a diamond shape (thumb to thumb and index finger to index finger).

2. Walk your feet back until your body is slightly inclined. Keep your feet positioned close together, preferably shoulder-width apart or slightly narrower, to maintain a stable base during the exercise.

3. Inhale, bend your elbows and lower your body towards the wall while maintaining a straight line from head to heels.

4. Exhale, straighten your arms and push your body back to the starting position.

5. Repeat for the recommended number of repetitions and sets.

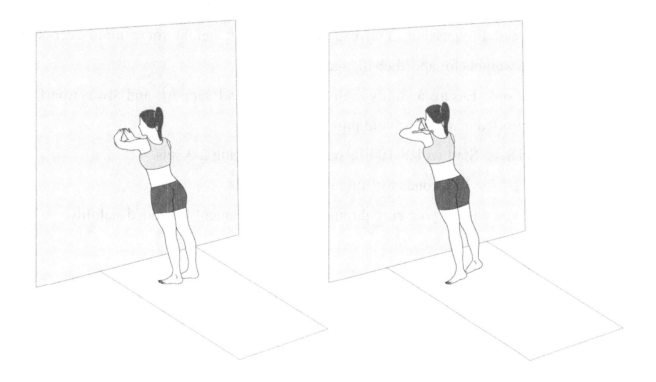

Wall Single-Leg Lift

• Target Muscle: Glutes, Hamstrings.

• Who Can Do It: Suitable for everyone, particularly beneficial for strengthening their lower body. Consult with a healthcare professional before starting a new exercise routine.

• Benefits: Helps strengthen the glutes and hamstrings and improves lower body strength, balance, and coordination.

• Form and Alignment Tips: Stand facing the wall. The body is bent at a 90-degree angle. Press your hands against the wall. Then move your right leg to the side.

• Common Mistakes to Avoid: Avoid hyperextending your back or swinging your leg. Movement should be controlled.

• Breathing: Inhale as you lift your leg, exhale as you lower your leg.

• Modification and Progression: You can reduce the lift height for a more accessible version or add ankle weights for added challenge.

• Safety Precautions: Ensure a sturdy wall for balance and support, and always perform movements in a controlled manner to avoid injury.

• Repetition and Sets: Start with 8-10 lifts per leg, performing 2-3 sets.

• Rest Period: Rest for 30 seconds to 1 minute between sets.

• Notes: Ensure you engage your core throughout the movement for added stability.

Instructions:

1. Stand a couple of feet away from a wall. Bend at the waist to form an angle of about 90 degrees with your body. Extend your arms straight and place them on the wall, keeping a straight line from your arms to your upper body.

2. Inhale as you move your right leg to the side and extend it as far as possible.

3. Exhale, slowly lower your leg back to the starting position.

4. Repeat this for the suggested number of repetitions before switching to the other leg. Perform the recommended number of sets.

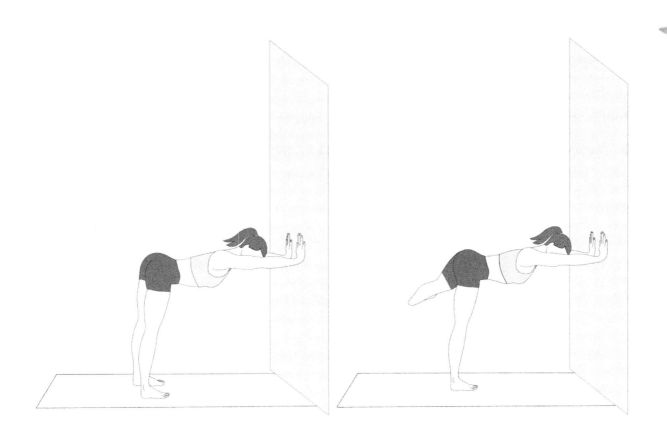

Wall Supported Warrior III Pose

- Target Muscle: Glutes, Hamstrings, Core.

- Who Can Do It: Suitable for everyone, particularly beneficial for improving balance, stability, and core strength. Always consult with a healthcare professional before beginning a new exercise routine.

- Benefits: Improves balance, strengthens the core and lower body, and aids posture correction.

- Form and Alignment Tips: Stand facing the wall, hands flat against the wall, and lean forward. Extend one leg behind you, creating a straight line from your head to your extended foot.

- Common Mistakes to Avoid: Avoid arching your back or swinging the extended leg. Make sure to keep the movement controlled and the body aligned.

- Breathing: Inhale as you lift your leg and lean forward, exhale as you return to the starting position.

- Modification and Progression: For beginners, reduce the lift height of the leg. You can lift the leg as you advance, eventually removing hand support.

- Safety Precautions: Make enough space around you to extend your leg and ensure the wall is sturdy.

- Repetition and Sets: Hold the pose for 30 seconds per side and perform 2-3 sets.

- Rest Period: Rest for 30 seconds to 1 minute between sets.

- Notes: Engage your core and glutes throughout the movement to maintain balance and stability.

Instructions:

1. Stand facing the wall, place both hands flat on the wall at shoulder height and slightly wider than shoulder-width apart.

2. Inhale as you lean forward, lifting one leg straight behind you.

3. Keep your body, arms, and the lifted leg straight. Hold this position, ensuring you maintain balance and form.

4. Exhale as you slowly lower your leg back to the starting position.

5. Repeat this process for the recommended number of breaths before switching to the other leg. Perform the suggested number of sets.

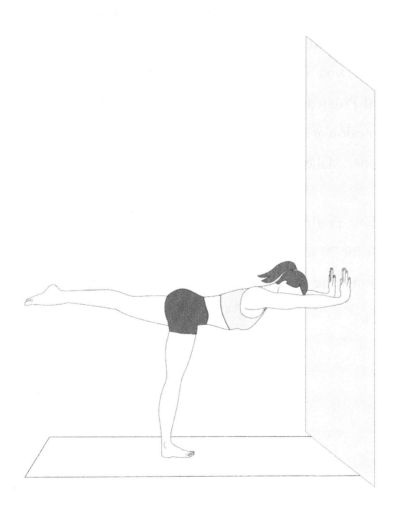

Wall Standing Side Kick

• Target Muscle: Glutes (gluteus medius and gluteus minimus), Outer Thighs (tensor fasciae latae).

• Who Can Do It: Suitable for everyone, especially beneficial for those looking to strengthen their glutes and outer thighs. Always consult with a healthcare professional before starting any new exercise routine.

• Benefits: Strengthens the glutes and outer thighs and improves hip mobility and balance.

• Form and Alignment Tips: Stand up straight and hold onto the wall with one hand for balance. Keep your moving leg straight during the kick and focus on engaging your glutes.

• Common Mistakes to Avoid: Avoid leaning too much into the wall or swinging the leg uncontrollably. The motion should be controlled and deliberate.

• Breathing: Inhale as you lift your leg to the side, exhale as you bring it back down.

• Modification and Progression: To modify and reduce the range of motion. To progress, increase the range of motion or add ankle weights.

• Safety Precautions: Make sure the wall is sturdy and has enough space to perform the exercise.

• Repetition and Sets: Perform 10-15 kicks per side for 2-3 sets.

• Rest Period: Rest for 30 seconds to 1 minute between sets.

• Notes: Engage your core for balance and to ensure your glutes and not momentum drive the movement.

Instructions:

1. Stand upright and place one hand on the wall for balance. Bend the other arm slightly and touch the side of your torso with the hand for better balance.
2. Slowly lift your leg straight to the side, while keeping your body straight.
3. Inhale as you lift your leg to the side hold for a second at the top.
4. Exhale and slowly lower your leg back to the starting position.
5. Repeat for the recommended number of repetitions and then switch to the other leg.
6. Perform the suggested number of sets.

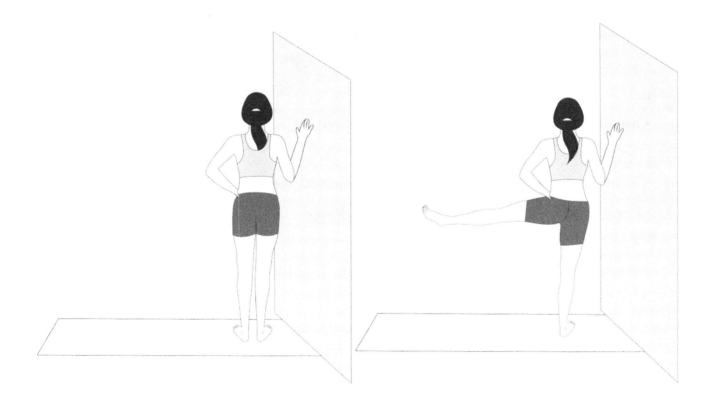

Wall Sit

• Target Muscle: Quadriceps, Glutes, Calves, Core.

• Who Can Do It: Suitable for individuals of all fitness levels, especially beneficial for those working on their lower body and core strength.

• Benefits: Increases endurance and strength in the lower body, particularly the quadriceps. It helps improve core stability.

• Form and Alignment Tips: Maintain a 90-degree angle at your knees and keep your back flat against the wall. Engage your core and keep your hands by your sides or before you.

• Common Mistakes to Avoid: Avoid sliding down too low or letting your knees go past your toes. Keep your knees in line with your ankles.

• Breathing: Inhale before you descend into the wall, sit, and exhale while you hold the position.

• Modification and Progression: To modify, hold for a shorter duration. To progress, keep for a longer time.

• Safety Precautions: Make sure the wall is sturdy, and you have a non-slip floor.

• Repetition and Sets: Hold the position for 20-60 seconds, for 2-3 sets.

• Rest Period: Rest for 30 seconds to 1 minute between sets.

• Notes: If discomfort is felt in the knees, leave the position and reset.

Instructions:

1. Stand about 1 foot from the wall and lean back to press your back flat against it.

2. Slide down the wall until your knees are bent at a 90-degree angle. Keep your thighs parallel to the floor.

3. Press your back flat into the wall, engage your core, and keep your hands by your sides or in front of you.

4. Hold this position, remembering to breathe evenly.

5. Push back up to the starting position to rest before the next set or to finish the exercise.

6. Repeat for the suggested number of sets.

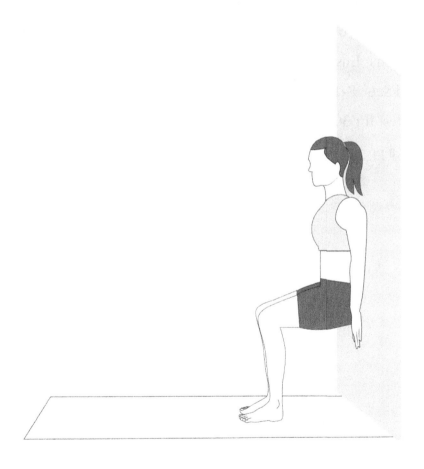

Wall Split Squats

• Target Muscle: Quadriceps, Hamstrings, Glutes.

• Who Can Do It: Suitable for intermediate and advanced fitness levels. Beneficial for those looking to improve lower body strength and stability.

• Benefits: This exercise effectively targets the quadriceps, hamstrings, and glutes, improving balance and flexibility.

• Form and Alignment Tips: You should stand on one leg with your back to the wall. The other leg should be bent at a 90-degree angle. Its foot should be leaning against the wall.

• Common Mistakes to Avoid: Don't allow your front knee to extend past your toes. Keep your back straight and avoid leaning forward.

• Breathing: Inhale as you lower the squat, exhale as you push up to standing.

• Safety Precautions: Ensure the floor is not slippery to prevent balance loss.

• Repetition and Sets: 8-12 repetitions on each leg for 2-3 sets.

• Rest Period: Rest for 30-60 seconds between sets.

• Notes: Ensure a proper warm-up before performing this exercise to avoid injuries.

Instructions:

1. Stand facing away from the wall. Position one foot flat against the wall, with the knee bent at a 90-degree angle. Plant the other foot firmly on the ground about 2 feet in front.

2. Position your hands behind your head.

3. Bend the knee of your front leg and lower your body toward the ground, keeping the chest upright and the core engaged.

4. Lower until your front thigh is almost parallel to the ground, ensuring your front knee doesn't extend past your toes.

5. Push through the front foot to rise back up to the starting position.

6. Repeat for the suggested number of repetitions, then switch legs.

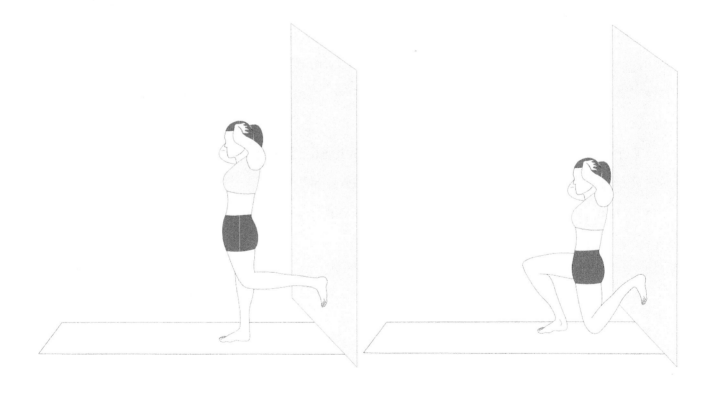

Wall-Supported One-Leg Squat

• Target Muscle: Quadriceps, Glutes, Hamstrings.

• Who Can Do It: Ideal for individuals with an intermediate fitness level. Those looking to improve lower body strength and balance can particularly benefit.

• Benefits: This exercise targets and strengthens the quads, glutes, and hamstrings, improving single-leg strength, balance, and mobility.

• Form and Alignment Tips: Keep your back flat against the wall. Ensure the knee of your working leg doesn't extend past your toes. Maintain an upright posture.

• Common Mistakes to Avoid: Avoid leaning too forward and keep the non-working leg straight during the movement.

• Breathing: Inhale as you lower the squat, exhale as you push back up to standing.

• Modification and Progression: Beginners can use a lower range of motion or perform a two-legged squat. For progression, try the exercise without wall support.

• Safety Precautions: Start with a smaller range of motion to ensure you can maintain balance and control.

• Repetition and Sets: 6-8 repetitions on each leg for 2-3 sets.

• Rest Period: Rest for 30-60 seconds between sets.

• Notes: Take your time with this exercise. Concentrate on maintaining balance and proper form.

Instructions:

1. Stand with your back against the wall. Position your feet hip-width apart.

2. Raise one leg in front of you, keeping it straight.

3. Lower into a squat on the supporting leg while raising the other leg, ensuring your back remains flat against the wall and your hands are along your sides for balance. Lower until the thigh of the squatting leg is parallel to the floor or as far as you can comfortably go.

4. Push through the foot to rise back to the standing position.

5. Repeat for the suggested number of repetitions, then switch legs.

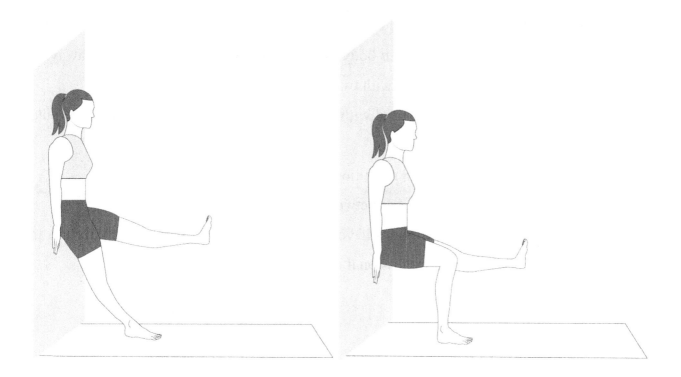

Wall-Assisted Single-Arm Push-Up

• Target Muscle: Chest, Shoulders, Triceps.

• Who Can Do It: This exercise suits intermediate to advanced fitness levels. It progresses from regular push-ups and requires good upper-body strength and balance.

• Benefits: Strengthens the chest, shoulders, and triceps, as well as engaging the core muscles for stability. It can enhance unilateral strength and balance.

• Form and Alignment Tips: Keep your body in a straight line from head to heels. Maintain a slight bend in your elbow of the supporting arm to avoid hyperextension. Ensure the working arm's shoulders, elbow, and wrist are aligned in the press position.

• Common Mistakes to Avoid: Avoid locking out your elbow fully or sagging in the hips.

• Breathing: Inhale as you lower your body towards the wall, exhale as you push away.

• Modification: Beginners can start with two-handed wall push-ups.

• Safety Precautions: Start slowly and with control to prevent undue stress on the shoulder joint.

• Repetition and Sets: Aim for 5-8 repetitions per arm for 2-3 sets.

• Rest Period: Rest for 30-60 seconds between sets.

• Notes: Always listen to your body. If you feel discomfort in your shoulder, return to a two-handed version and consult a professional if needed.

Instructions:

1. Stand arm's length away from a wall, facing towards it.

2. Place one palm flat against the wall, aligning it with your chest. Keep your arm slightly bent.

3. Keep the other hand behind your back.

4. Lower your chest towards the wall by bending your elbow.

5. Push your body away from the wall, extending your arm to return to the start position.

6. Repeat for the suggested number of repetitions, then switch arms.

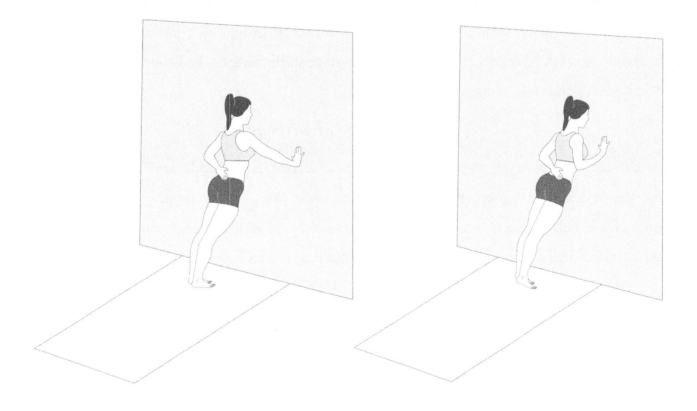

Chapter 7: The 28-Day Challenge

The human body is a marvel of design and engineering. We're made to move, and with consistent training and the right exercises, we can push our physical limits to heights we never thought possible. It's our pleasure to present you with this 28-day fitness plan constructed to do exactly that.

The 28-day plan is designed to take you on a journey from beginner to advanced+ in just four weeks, focusing on bodyweight exercises that utilize a wall as the primary support.

Why this plan is good for you:

This plan allows you to work out in the comfort of your home, using only your body weight and a wall, making it both convenient and accessible. The exercises have been chosen to provide a full-body workout, targeting all major muscle groups and promoting strength and flexibility. Moreover, these exercises help improve posture, balance, and coordination, vital for overall health and well-being.

How to execute this plan:

Each day is structured with a warm-up, main exercises, rest periods, and a cool-down. The warm-up is designed to prepare your body and mind for the workout, reduce the risk of injury, and increase performance. Rest periods are essential for muscle recovery and growth. Lastly, cooling down helps return your heart rate to normal and reduce muscle stiffness post-workout.

Performing each exercise properly is essential to maximize effectiveness and prevent injuries.

Remember, consistency is critical. Please stick to the plan even when it's tough; you will see improvements. Every single repetition is a step toward your goal. Don't compare your day 1 to someone else's day 28. This is your journey, and every effort you make counts.

Notes

Listen to your body. If an exercise feels too difficult, modify it to your level, or decrease the number of repetitions/sets. If you experience pain (beyond typical muscle fatigue), stop the exercise. Rest is just as important as the workout for muscle recovery and growth. Hydrate, maintain a balanced diet, and get adequate sleep.

Finally, consult with a healthcare professional before starting any new fitness program, especially if you have pre-existing health conditions.

Embrace the challenge, stay committed, and, most importantly, enjoy the process. Your journey to fitness starts now. Good luck!

Remember, the goal of this plan is not just about looking better but feeling better, having more energy, and leading a healthier, more fulfilling life. You can make a positive change, and this book is your guide to doing just that. Let's get started!

DAY 1

Name	Note	Page number
Warm-Up	5 minutes	15
Wall Plank	2 sets of 20-30 seconds hold	20
Wall Supported Warrior III Pose	2 sets of 30 seconds per side	66
Wall Arm Circles	2 sets of 10-15 circles	42
Wall Single Leg Lift	2 sets of 8-10 reps per leg	64
Cool-Down	5 minutes of stretching	17

DAY 2

Name	Note	Page number
Warm-Up	5 minutes	15
Wall-Assisted Knees Side to Side	2 sets of 10-12 reps per side	26
Wall Triceps Dips	2 sets of 10-12 reps	38
Wall Abdominal Crunches	2 sets of 10-12 reps	56
Wall Roll-Down	2 sets of 8-10 reps	24
Cool-Down	5 minutes of stretching	17

DAY 3

Name	Note	Page number
Warm-Up	5 minutes	15
Wall Leg Circles	2 sets of 15 circles per leg	32
Single Leg Balance	2 sets of 15-20 seconds hold per side	44
Wall-Assisted Lunges	2 sets of 8-10 reps per leg	52
Wall Assisted Single Arm Push-Up	2 sets of 6-8 reps per arm	76
Cool-Down	5 minutes of stretching	17

DAY 4

Name	Note	Page number
Warm-Up	5 minutes	15
Wall Lateral Pull Downs	2 sets of 12-15 reps	40
Wall Mountain Climbers	2 sets of 20 reps (10 per leg)	46
Wall-Assisted Diamond Push-Ups	2 sets of 10-12 reps	62
Wall Bridge	2 sets of 30 sec	48
Cool-Down	5 minutes of stretching	17

DAY 5

Name	Note	Page number
Warm-Up	5 minutes	15
Wall Arm Circles	2 sets of 10-15 circles	42
Wall Marches	2 sets of 20 reps (10 per leg)	28
Wall Supported One-Leg Squat	2 sets of 6-8 reps per leg	74
Wall-Assisted Squat (Sliding)	2 sets of 10-12 reps	58
Cool-Down	5 minutes of stretching	17

DAY 6

Name	Note	Page number
Warm-Up	5 minutes	15
Wall Leg Extension	2 sets of 8-10 reps	60
Wall Scissor Kicks	2 sets of 12-15 reps	50
Wall Single Leg Bridge	2 sets of 10-12 reps per leg	54
Wall Sit	2 sets of 30 seconds hold	70
Cool-Down	5 minutes of stretching	17

(DAY 7 - REST) DAY 8

Name	Note	Page number
Warm-Up	5 minutes	15
Wall Plank	2 sets of 20-30 seconds hold	20
Wall Supported Warrior III Pose	2 sets of 30 seconds per side	66
Wall Arm Circles	2 sets of 20 circles	42
Wall Single Leg Lift	2 sets of 10-12 reps per leg	64
Cool-Down	5 minutes of stretching	17

DAY 9

Name	Note	Page number
Warm-Up	5 minutes	15
Wall-Assisted Knees Side to Side	2 sets of 12-15 reps per side	26
Wall Push-Ups	2 sets of 10-15 reps	36
Wall Triceps Dips	2 sets of 12-15 reps	38
Wall Roll-Down	2 sets of 10-12 reps	24
Cool-Down	5 minutes of stretching	17

DAY 10

Name	Note	Page number
Warm-Up	5 minutes	15
Wall Leg Circles	2 sets of 15 circles per leg	32
Single Leg Balance	2 sets of 20-30 seconds hold per side	44
Wall-Assisted Lunges	2 sets of 10-12 reps per leg	52
Wall-Assisted Single-Arm Push-Up	2 sets of 8-10 reps per arm	76
Cool-Down	5 minutes of stretching	17

DAY 11

Name	Note	Page number
Warm-Up	5 minutes	15
Wall Lateral Pull Downs	2 sets of 12-15 reps	40
Wall Mountain Climbers	2 sets of 20 reps (10 per leg)	46
Wall-Assisted Diamond Push-Ups	2 sets of 12-15 reps	62
Wall Leg Extension	2 sets of 12-15 reps	60
Cool-Down	5 minutes of stretching	17

DAY 12

Name	Note	Page number
Warm-Up	5 minutes	15
Wall Arm Circles	2 sets of 20 circles	42
Wall Marches	2 sets of 30 reps (15 per leg)	28
Wall Supported One-Leg Squat	2 sets of 6-8 reps per leg	74
Wall-Assisted Squat (Sliding)	2 sets of 12-15 reps	58
Cool-Down	5 minutes of stretching	17

DAY 13

Name	Note	Page number
Warm-Up	5 minutes	15
Wall Glute Kickbacks	2 sets of 10-15 reps per leg	30
Wall Scissor Kicks	2 sets of 15-17 reps	50
Wall Single Leg Bridge	2 sets of 12-15 reps per leg	54
Wall Sit	2 sets of 30-45 seconds hold	70
Cool-Down	5 minutes of stretching	17

(DAY 14 - REST) DAY 15

Name	Note	Page number
Warm-Up	5 minutes	15
Wall Plank	2 sets of 30-45 seconds hold	20
Wall Supported Warrior III Pose	2 sets of 30-45 seconds per side	66
Wall Arm Circles	2 sets of 25 circles	42
Wall Single Leg Lift	2 sets of 12-15 reps per leg	64
Cool-Down	5 minutes of stretching	17

DAY 16

Name	Note	Page number
Warm-Up	5 minutes	15
Wall-Assisted Knees Side to Side	2 sets of 12-15 reps per side	26
Wall Push-Ups	2 sets of 12-15 reps	36
Wall Triceps Dips	2 sets of 12-15 reps	38
Wall Roll-Down	2 sets of 12-15 reps	24
Cool-Down	5 minutes of stretching	17

DAY 17

Name	Note	Page number
Warm-Up	5 minutes	15
Wall Leg Circles	2 sets of 20 circles per leg	32
Single Leg Balance	2 sets of 20-30 seconds hold per side	44
Wall-Assisted Lunges	2 sets of 10-12 reps per leg	52
Wall-Assisted Single-Arm Push-Up	2 sets of 10-12 reps per arm	76
Cool-Down	5 minutes of stretching	17

DAY 18

Name	Note	Page number
Warm-Up	5 minutes	15
Wall Lateral Pull Downs	2 sets of 15-17 reps	40
Wall Mountain Climbers	2 sets of 30 reps (15 per leg)	46
Wall-Assisted Diamond Push-Ups	2 sets of 17-20 reps	62
Wall Leg Extension	2 sets of 12-15 reps	60
Cool-Down	5 minutes of stretching	17

DAY 19

Name	Note	Page number
Warm-Up	5 minutes	15
Wall Arm Circles	2 sets of 30 circles	42
Wall Marches	2 sets of 40 reps (20 per leg)	28
Wall Push-Ups	2 sets of 12-15 reps	36
Wall Sit	2 sets of 30-45 seconds hold	70
Cool-Down	5 minutes of stretching	17

DAY 20

Name	Note	Page number
Warm-Up	5 minutes	15
Wall Leg Extension	2 sets of 15-17 reps	60
Wall Scissor Kicks	2 sets of 17-20 reps	50
Wall Single Leg Bridge	2 sets of 15-17 reps per leg	54
Wall Standing Side Kick	2 sets of 15 reps per leg	68
Cool-Down	5 minutes of stretching	17

(DAY 21 - REST) DAY 22

Name	Note	Page number
Warm-Up	5 minutes	15
Wall Plank	2 sets of 30-45 seconds hold	20
Wall Supported Warrior III Pose	2 sets of 45 seconds per side	66
Wall Arm Circles	2 sets of 30 circles	42
Single Leg Balance	2 sets of 30-45 seconds hold per side	44
Cool-Down	5 minutes of stretching	17

DAY 23

Name	Note	Page number
Warm-Up	5 minutes	15
Wall Roll-Down	2 sets of 15-17 reps	24
Wall Push-Ups	2 sets of 15-17 reps	36
Wall Glute Kickbacks	2 sets of 12-15 reps per leg	30
Wall-Assisted Knees Side to Side	2 sets of 15-17 reps per side	26
Cool-Down	5 minutes of stretching	17

DAY 24

Name	Note	Page number
Warm-Up	5 minutes	15
Wall Leg Circlcs	2 sets of 25 circles per leg	32
Single Leg Balance	2 sets of 30-45 seconds hold per side	44
Wall-Assisted Lunges	2 sets of 12-15 reps per leg	52
Wall Calf Raises	2 sets of 15-20 reps	34
Cool-Down	5 minutes of stretching	17

DAY 25

Name	Note	Page number
Warm-Up	5 minutes	15
Wall Abdominal Crunches	2 sets of 12-15 reps	56
Wall Mountain Climbers	2 sets of 40 reps (20 per leg)	46
Wall-Assisted Diamond Push-Ups	2 sets of 20 reps	62
Wall-Assisted Bridge	2-3 sets of 10-15 reps	22
Cool-Down	5 minutes of stretching	17

(DAY 26 - REST) DAY 27

Name	Note	Page number
Warm-Up	5 minutes	15
Wall Glute Kickbacks	2 sets of 15-20 reps per leg	30
Wall Scissor Kicks	2 sets of 20 reps	50
Wall Single Leg Bridge	2 sets of 17-20 reps per leg	54
Wall Sit	2 sets of 60 seconds hold	70
Cool-Down	5 minutes of stretching	17

DAY 28

Name	Note	Page number
Warm-Up	5 minutes	15
Wall-Assisted Knees Side to Side	2 sets of 20 reps per side	26
Wall Push-Ups	2 sets of 20 reps	36
Wall-Assisted Bridge	2-3 sets of 10-15 reps	22
Wall Roll-Down	2 sets of 20 reps	24
Cool-Down	5 minutes of stretching	17

Bonus Chapter: Mindfulness and Breathing Techniques in Wall Pilates

As we embark on this journey into the heart of Wall Pilates, it's imperative to underscore two critical components of this practice - mindfulness and breathing techniques. The interplay of these elements elevates Wall Pilates beyond just another form of exercise, transforming it into a holistic approach that enhances both your physical fitness and mental well-being.

Some may ask, "*Why is mindfulness important in Wall Pilates?*" The answer lies in the essence of Pilates itself. Unlike other fitness regimes that focus solely on physical intensity, Pilates engages both your body and mind, fostering a deep connection between the two. It calls for your unwavering attention to each movement, requiring you to be fully present in the moment. This emphasis on mindfulness helps to hone your body awareness, improve focus, and reduce stress.

Likewise, breathing techniques hold immense significance in Wall Pilates. Proper breathing fuels your body with the necessary oxygen and facilitates better movement and core engagement. It synchronizes your mind with your body's rhythms, intensifying your workouts while promoting relaxation and stress relief.

This chapter will unravel the intricacies of mindfulness and breathing techniques in Wall Pilates. These skills will amplify your Wall Pilates practice and positively impact your daily life, bringing clarity, calmness, and control. So, let's get started on this enlightening journey.

Understanding Mindfulness

Mindfulness is the practice of focusing on the present moment without judgment. Instead of being swept away by thoughts about the past or future, we bring our attention back to the here and now. By applying mindfulness to Wall Pilates, you can enhance your mind-body connection, increase your concentration, and improve the effectiveness of each workout.

Practicing Mindfulness in Wall Pilates

Body Scan: This is a simple yet effective practice to bring awareness to your body and prepare for the workout.

Step-by-Step Instructions:

1. Start by closing your eyes and taking deep breaths.
2. Begin to scan your body from your head to your toes mentally.
3. Pay attention to any sensations, tensions, or areas of relaxation.
4. Try to observe without judgment or the urge to change anything.
5. The goal is to become more attuned to your body's state before you exercise.

Single-Tasking: Doing just one thing at a time can be incredibly powerful in a world that glorifies multitasking. When you're working out, focus on the exercise at hand.

Tips: If your mind drifts off, gently guide your attention to your movements and breath. It's perfectly normal for the mind to wander, but the practice lies in bringing it back each time.

Mastering Breathing Techniques in Wall Pilates

Proper breathing is a fundamental part of Wall Pilates, as it helps to stabilize your core, improve your movements' precision, and enhance your overall performance.

Lateral Breathing: This is the primary breathing technique used in Pilates, and it involves inhaling and exhaling deeply without disturbing the position of the chest and shoulders.

Step-by-Step Instructions:

1. Sit or stand in a comfortable position.
2. Place your hands on the sides of your rib cage.
3. Inhale through your nose, focusing on expanding your rib cage sideways as if you're trying to push your hands apart.
4. Exhale through your mouth, feel your rib cage contract, and pull your belly button towards your spine.
5. Practice this technique for a few minutes each day until it becomes second nature.

Breath Pacing: Coordinating your breath with your movements can help you to perform exercises more effectively and maintain a rhythm throughout your workout.

Tips: If you find it challenging to sync your breathing with your movements, don't worry! With practice, it will become more intuitive. To start, inhaling during the preparation phase of an exercise and exhaling during the exertion phase.

Remember, the essence of Pilates lies in the harmonious coordination of breath, movement, and mindfulness. By consciously integrating these elements into your routine, you'll strengthen your body and cult Advanced Mindfulness Techniques in Wall Pilates.

Beyond the body scan and single-tasking, you can use more advanced mindfulness techniques to deepen your practice.

Moving with Intention: In Wall Pilates, every movement is deliberate and serves a purpose. Bringing an element of intentionality to your exercises can enhance your focus and result in a more effective workout.

Step-by-Step Instructions:

1. Before you begin each exercise, take a moment to prepare mentally.
2. Visualize the movements you're about to perform and how your body will feel as you do them.
3. As you move, remember every contraction, extension, and release.

Cultivating Non-Judgmental Awareness: Being mindful means observing without judging. This practice can help you avoid self-criticism during workouts and build a more positive relationship with your body.

Tips: When you notice judgmental thoughts creeping in, gently acknowledge them and then let them go. Remind yourself that you're not here to achieve perfection but to improve a little bit every day.

Advanced Breathing Techniques in Wall Pilates

You can incorporate more advanced breathing techniques into your routine as you become more comfortable with lateral breathing and breath pacing.

Coordinated Breathing: Coordinating your breath with your movements more precisely can help you perform exercises more efficiently and control your body's movements better.

Step-by-Step Instructions:

1. Take the "Wall Roll Down" exercise as an example.

2. Start standing upright against the wall.

3. As you exhale, slowly roll your spine away from the wall, vertebra by vertebra, until you're in a forward bend. Pause here and inhale.

4. As you exhale, slowly roll back up to the starting position. The exhalation guides the movement, and the inhalation serves as a moment of rest.

   Breath Control: Gaining more control over your breath can help you stabilize your core and enhance your overall performance.

Tips:

- Experiment with different breathing rhythms to see what works best.

- Try breathing in for a count of four, breathing out for six, or breathing in and out for equal counts.

- Find a rhythm that feels comfortable and sustainable for you.

- By combining these advanced techniques with the foundations of mindfulness and breathing in Wall Pilates, you can take your workouts to a new level. Remember, the ultimate goal is strengthening and toning your body and cultivating a calm, focused, and resilient mind.

Bonus Chapter: Nutrition Guide for Wall Pilates Practitioners

Understanding nutrition's critical role in our fitness journey is the first step toward creating a holistic and effective workout regimen. Regarding Wall Pilates, proper nutrition is equally important as the exercises themselves. A balanced diet provides the necessary fuel for your workouts and aids in quicker recovery and better overall health.

The Importance of Proper Nutrition:

While you engage your body in the invigorating practice of Wall Pilates, ensuring that your nutrition complements your efforts is vital. The right food choices can help:

Provide Energy: Our body needs adequate energy to perform exercises effectively. A well-balanced diet ensures a steady supply of energy, which can lead to more productive and intense workout sessions.

Aid Recovery: Physical activities like Wall Pilates induce muscle stress and inflammation. Nutrient-dense foods provide the essential vitamins and minerals that help in quicker recovery and muscle repair.

Enhance Overall Health: Combining exercise with balanced nutrition results in overall well-being, improved body composition, better mental health, and a robust immune system.

How to Incorporate Proper Nutrition:

Now that we understand why nutrition is essential let's discuss how to incorporate healthy eating habits into our daily routines. Here are some practical strategies:

Balanced Meals: Strive for a balanced diet rich in lean proteins, whole grains, fruits, vegetables, and healthy fats. Each food group plays a distinct role in our body and contributes to our fitness differently.

Pre-workout Meals: Eating a light, balanced meal or snack about 2 hours before your Wall Pilates session is crucial. This timing ensures that your body has had adequate time to digest the food and convert it into energy for your workout. Foods like bananas, yogurt, oats, or a smoothie can be excellent choices to provide you with the necessary power.

Post-workout Nutrition: Your body starts to recover once your workout is finished. It requires nutrients, particularly protein, and carbohydrates, to repair muscles and replenish depleted energy stores. For protein-rich foods, consider choices like lean meats (chicken, turkey), eggs, and beans, and for carbohydrates, think about options such as brown rice, whole wheat bread, potatoes, and fruits like apples and berries. Consuming a meal or snack with these macronutrients within an hour after your session is essential to promote efficient recovery and muscle growth.

Mindful Eating: Paying attention to your hunger and fullness cues, savoring each bite, and reducing distraction while eating can significantly improve your relationship with food and contribute to better nutritional habits.

Nutrition is a broad and complex topic; these are just basic guidelines. Individual needs can significantly vary based on age, sex, weight, medical conditions, and the intensity of workouts. Consider consulting a registered dietitian or nutrition professional for more personalized advice.

Hydration

Proper hydration is integral to our overall health and optimizing our fitness endeavors, especially when partaking in intense exercises like Wall Pilates. Delving into its significance reveals:

Cellular Function and Metabolism: Every cell relies on water. Water plays an indispensable role in generating energy and fostering muscle development, from driving essential biochemical reactions to aiding nutrient absorption, digestion, and metabolism.

Joint Lubrication: Consistent hydration ensures that our joint cartilage retains its necessary moisture, enabling smoother and less strenuous movements during workouts.

Temperature Regulation: When we exert ourselves physically, our bodies generate heat. Water's role in heat dissipation, primarily through sweating, is crucial to prevent overheating and sustain more extended and efficient workouts.

Detoxification: Effective kidney function, critical for flushing toxins and waste, hinges on proper hydration. Removing these waste products helps stave off fatigue and ensures a steady energy output during workouts.

Skin Health: A well-hydrated body often reflects in the quality of one's skin. Water assists in preserving skin elasticity, warding off dryness, and promoting a luminous complexion.

Enhanced Physical Performance: Hydration bolsters muscle function, diminishes the likelihood of cramps and sustains stamina and strength, all pivotal in any fitness journey.

The quantity of water one should consume often correlates with body weight. Generally, a recommendation is to drink at least 30 to 35 ml of water for every kilogram of body weight. For example, a woman weighing 60 kilograms might aim to consume 1.8 to 2.1 liters of water daily. However, this can vary based on physical activity, ambient temperature, and individual health considerations.

Yet, the balance remains essential. Overconsumption of water in a brief span can lead to conditions like water intoxication or hyponatremia, which can strain the kidneys and be potentially harmful.

To align with optimal hydration guidelines, consider drinking about 500 ml (17 ounces) of water 2 to 3 hours before your Wall Pilates session, complemented by an additional 250 ml (8 ounces) about 20 to 30 minutes pre-workout. Sipping water regularly during the session helps in sustaining hydration levels.

Being in tune with your body's cues is vital. Often, when we feel thirsty, our bodies have already started experiencing the early stages of dehydration. Thus, a proactive approach to hydration throughout the day is recommended.

In conclusion, proper nutrition can significantly impact your Wall Pilates journey. It fuels your body, aids in recovery, and helps you achieve your fitness goals more effectively. So, as you embrace the empowering practice of Wall Pilates, let's also commit to fueling our bodies with the nutritious food it deserves. Remember, health and fitness are not just about how much you can lift or how flexible you are but also about how well you nourish your body.

Conclusion

As we reach the final pages of this book, we have navigated the inspiring world of Wall Pilates together, uncovering its many facets. We have explored the practicalities of setting up your practice space, understanding and performing warm-ups, maintaining proper form, and choosing practical exercises. We've delved into the significant realms of mindfulness and breathing techniques, emphasizing their intrinsic role in Wall Pilates and overall wellness. Additionally, we've highlighted the impact of nutritional choices on your Pilates performance and well-being.

Now, the knowledge is in your hands. The path to fitness, balance, and well-being is laid before you, and it's time to step forward. Take this newly acquired knowledge, these tools, and techniques, and integrate them into your daily routine. The transformation you seek starts with action.

Thank you for accompanying me on this Wall Pilates journey. Your commitment to learning and improving your health is commendable. If you've found value and guidance in this book, please leave a review on Amazon. Your insights can be the beacon that guides others on their wellness journey.

And now, as we close this chapter, another one opens in your life - your personal Wall Pilates journey. Revel in the challenges, savor the progress, and trust your capacity to evolve. As this book concludes, remember your journey is just beginning. Here's to a healthier, stronger, and more balanced you.

ABOUT THE AUTHOR

Emily Lemberg wears many hats, but her roles as a dedicated yoga and Pilates instructor stand out the most. For years, she has been an advocate for harnessing both disciplines' strength and serenity. Her passion lies in guiding individuals to discover the transformative power of these practices, especially in the bustling whirlwind of modern life.

In "Wall Pilates Workouts for Women," Emily unveils a fresh perspective on Pilates. By integrating the wall into traditional routines, she presents a method that's both innovative and accessible. This book is a testament to her commitment to making fitness and well-being achievable for everyone, regardless of age or experience level.

Emily's approach goes beyond just physical postures. She emphasizes the harmony between the mind, body, and spirit - a philosophy she embodies in her teachings and daily life.

Outside of her classes and writings, Emily finds joy in simple pleasures. She loves soaking up the tranquility of nature, delving into enlightening reads, and spending quality time with loved ones.

Workout Reflections

Made in the USA
Coppell, TX
14 October 2023